GLUTEN-FREE
BAKING

PHIL VICKERY

Photography by Tara

FIREFLY BOOKS

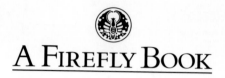

A FIREFLY BOOK

Published by Firefly Books Ltd. 2011

First printing

Publisher Cataloging-in-Publication Data (U.S.)

Vickery, Phil.
    Gluten-free baking / Phil Vickery.
[176] p. : ill., photos. (some col.) ; cm.
Includes index.
Summary: A collection of over 70 recipes designed
for those with gluten intolerance.
ISBN-13: 978-1-55407-811-0
ISBN-10: 1-55407-811-3
1. Gluten-free diet — Recipes. I. Title.
641.5638 dc22   RM237.86V535 2011

**Library and Archives Canada Cataloguing in
Publication**

Vickery, Phil
    Gluten-free baking / Phil Vickery.
Includes index.
ISBN-13: 978-1-55407-811-0
ISBN-10: 1-55407-811-3
    1. Gluten-free diet — Recipes. 2. Baking. I. Title.
RM237.86.V53 2011   641.5'638   C2010-906269-8

Published in the United States by
Firefly Books (U.S.) Inc.
P.O. Box 1338, Ellicott Station
Buffalo, New York 14205

Published in Canada by
Firefly Books Ltd.
66 Leek Crescent
Richmond Hill, Ontario L4B 1H1

Printed in China by C&C Offset Printing Co.

Developed by:
Kyle Cathie Limited
23 Howland Street, London W1T 4AY
general.enquiries@kyle-cathie.com
www.kylecathie.com

Project editor: Jenny Wheatley
Photographer: Tara Fisher
Designer: Jacqui Caulton
Food stylist: Annie Rigg
Props stylist: Wei Tang
Copy editor: Jane Bamforth
Editorial assistant: Elanor Clarke
Americanizer: Lee Faber
Production: Gemma John

GLUTEN-FREE
BAKING

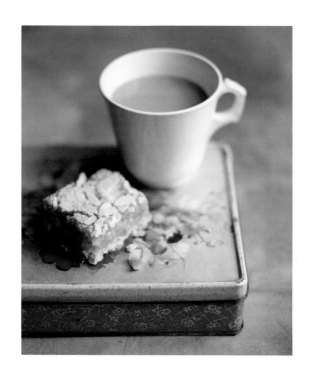

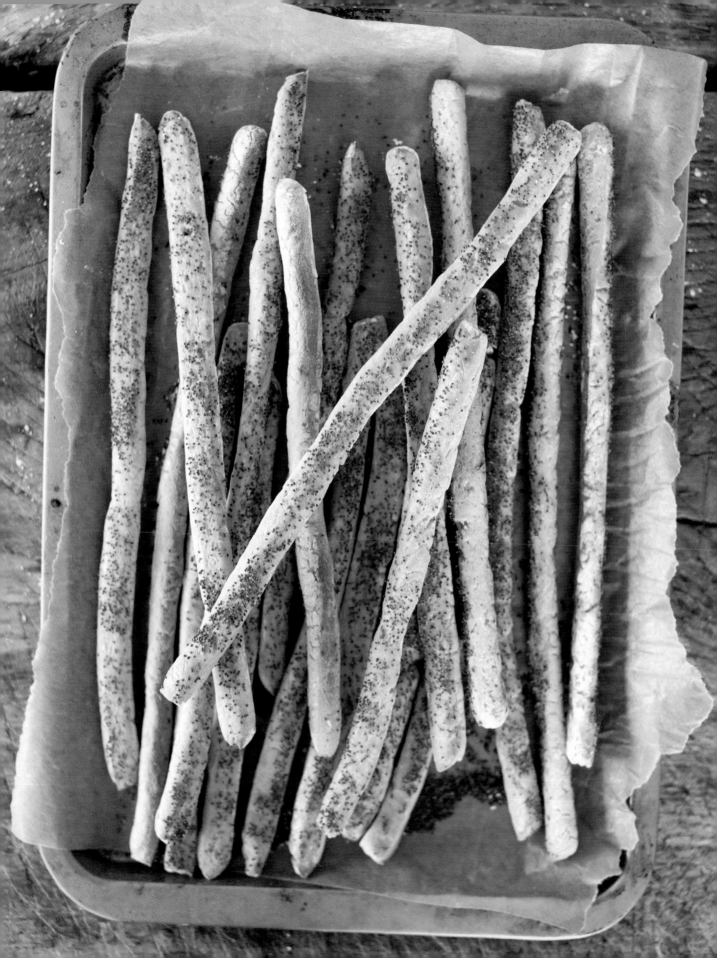

CONTENTS

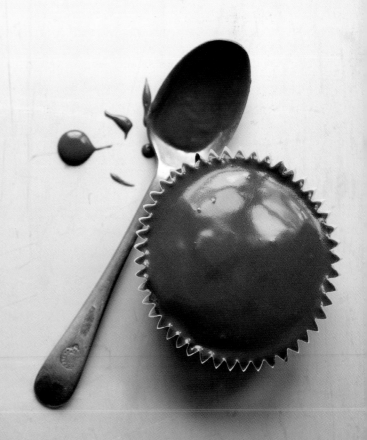

FOREWORD

When I decided to write *Seriously Good! Gluten-Free Cooking* a couple of years ago, it was after I'd started a gluten-free Christmas pudding company. The response to the puddings was so huge that I wanted to find out more about gluten-free diets. While researching, it quickly became apparent that celiac disease is a worldwide condition. So the idea to write a book dedicated to gluten-free cooking seemed like the obvious route to take.

People from all over the world have sent me e-mails and letters in response to the book. From moms who couldn't find a gluten-free birthday cake recipe for their kids, to a lady in her 90s, finally being able to eat "normal food" after 35 years with the condition—it's been a real eye-opener for me.

In the first book I covered all areas of cooking, with a section on desserts and baking. While the feedback has been incredible, the overwhelming themes were requests for gluten-free Yorkshire puddings, birthday cakes, Christmas cake, Welsh cakes, steamed puddings, sponge cakes, cupcakes, and of course bread!

So this book includes all of the above, plus new recipes for pastry, sheet cakes, muffins, cookies, and special occasion cakes. Also look out for some slightly unusual recipes: Tangy Beet and Black Currant Muffins, Sweet Zucchini and Saffron Butterfly Cakes, and Sweet Potato Thins all work really well, and certainly take gluten-free baking a step further.

It has taken me about a year to write this book, partly due to me writing slowly, but also due to the fact that it takes an incredible amount of time to cook and perfect each recipe. Sometimes a new idea works first time (great, but it didn't happen very often!); mostly, though, it has taken up to three, four, five, six, or even seven times to get it right! There have been many technical and scientific challenges to overcome to get the very best results each time, and I enlisted the help of my good friend, food scientist Bea Harling, to keep me on the straight and narrow. Her knowledge has been invaluable.

The final result is 70 recipes that I am very happy with. Some are far better, in my view, than conventional similar products, like the Vanilla Cupcakes for example. When it comes to bread, there will always be the inevitable comparison to regular bread; sadly you will never mimic it perfectly without many additives and chemicals, something that I try to steer clear of. But I'm really pleased with the recipes in the Bread chapter and urge you to have a go—whether it's focaccia, savory biscuits, or sweet breads, you'll discover that baking gluten-free bread truly can be rewarding.

I hope this book helps you in two ways: one, that it inspires you to get in the kitchen so you can discover how delicious gluten-free baking can be! And also that it helps to highlight celiac disease so that living on a gluten-free diet becomes easier in the future.

And finally, don't forget ...

People on a gluten-free diet can enjoy really delicious, flavorful food. In fact, a gluten-free diet not only offers the chance to improve the quality of the food you eat by cooking with fresh, unprocessed ingredients, but also helps to introduce your taste buds to new flavor combinations. The recipes in this book are all about expanding your gluten-free diet—giving you food to enjoy, food that is nutritious, and food that will make you feel ... seriously good!

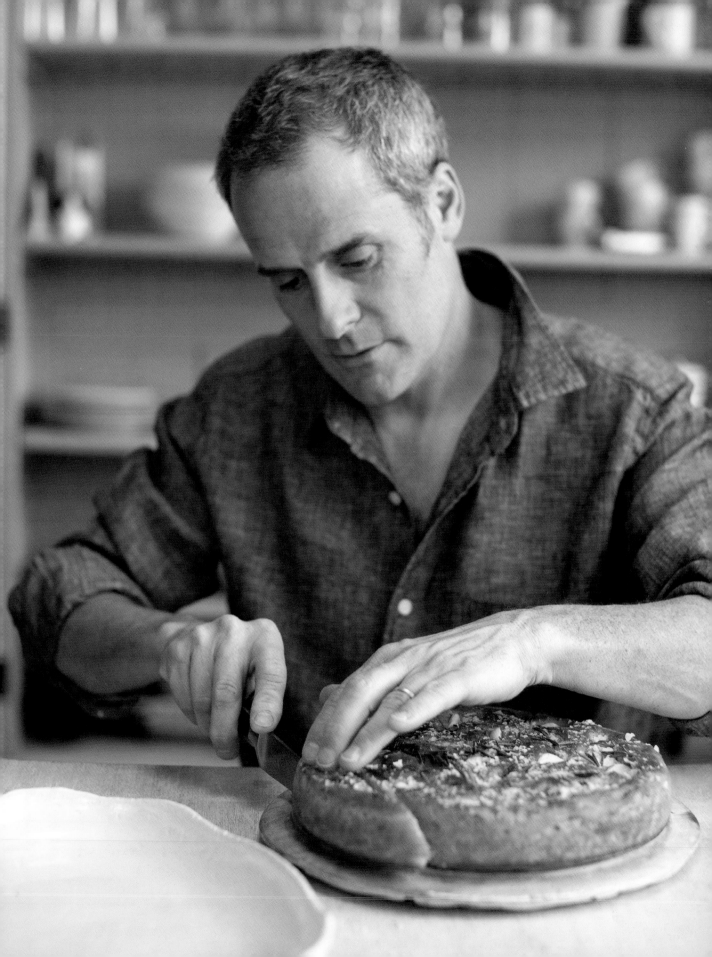

INTRODUCTION TO CELIAC DISEASE

If you have recently been diagnosed with celiac disease, don't panic—here are answers to the most commonly asked questions, along with advice on what to eat and what to avoid.

What is celiac disease?

Celiac (pronounced seeliac) disease is often misunderstood. It is frequently regarded as an allergy or simple food intolerance, but it is actually a lifelong autoimmune disease affecting the intestines and other parts of the body. The body's immune system reacts to the gluten found in food, making the body attack itself when gluten is eaten. Gluten is a protein found in wheat, barley, and rye, and some people are also affected by oats. Gluten is a collective name for the type of protein found in these cereals. It is what gives bread its elasticity and cakes their spring.

People with celiac disease are sensitive to gluten when it is eaten. The small intestine is lined with small, finger-like projections called villi. These play a crucial role in digestion, as they increase the surface area of the small intestine and allow essential nutrients to be absorbed into the bloodstream. However, for people with celiac disease, when gluten comes into contact with the villi, it triggers a response by the immune system that attacks the villi as if it were a "foreign" substance. The villi very quickly become damaged and inflamed, and therefore incapable of extracting key nutrients from the food we eat. This results in a range of different problems with varying severity.

What are the symptoms?

There is a variety of gastrointestinal symptoms, such as cramps, bloating, flatulence, and diarrhea. It is quite common for these to be confused with irritable bowel syndrome (IBS) and only later to be identified as celiac disease.

TYPICAL SYMPTOMS OF CELIAC DISEASE

The symptoms vary in terms of severity. Most stem from the malabsorption of nutrients and include diarrhea, fatigue, and iron deficiency, but there is a range of other symptoms, such as:

- Bloating
- Abdominal pains
- Nausea
- Tiredness
- Headaches
- Weight loss (but not in all cases)
- Mouth ulcers
- Hair loss
- Skin rash
- Defective tooth enamel
- Problems with fertility
- Recurrent miscarriages

Diarrhea is a common symptom. Yet it is important to note that sufferers can present many and varied symptoms: some may have a normal bowel habit, or even tend toward constipation, children may not gain weight or grow properly, while adults may find they lose weight. Malabsorption may also leave people tired and weak, due to anemia caused by iron deficiency.

In fact, rather than suffering from bowel problems, many people with celiac disease approach their doctor because of extreme tiredness (due to chronic, poor iron absorption) and psychological problems such as depression. There can also be a malabsorption of calcium, resulting in low bone density, and sometimes even fractures (as a result of osteoporosis). Bone and muscle pain can also be a problem. Ulcers in the mouth, or a blistering, itchy skin rash, mostly on the elbows and knees (called dermatitis herpetiformis), are also symptoms of celiac disease.

Undiagnosed celiac disease can result in infertility in both men and women, and there is also an increased risk of miscarriage.

How do I get diagnosed?

First, if you suspect you may have celiac disease, don't worry! Just remember, it is entirely manageable with a controlled diet. In fact, if you are one of the many undiagnosed people with celiac disease, you'll probably be pleased to find out that you really do have a condition, and, better yet, that there is a course of action to make you well again.

There is a clear procedure for diagnosing celiac disease. The first thing to do is talk through your symptoms with your doctor, as he or she can perform a simple blood test. This test looks for antibodies that your body produces in response to gluten. It is important to follow your normal diet leading up to the test, as you need to have the antibodies in your blood for a test to work, and these will only be there if you have been eating gluten. It is quite common for people to go undiagnosed if they have followed a gluten-free diet for days or weeks, as the immune system will be producing fewer antibodies. This will give a false negative result to the test. To get an accurate result, it is important to consume food that contains gluten in at least one meal a day for a minimum of six weeks before a blood test.

If the test is positive, it is recommended that people then have an intestinal biopsy, which examines the appearance of the villi in the small intestine under a microscope, to check for damage. This will confirm the diagnosis, which you need before you start on a lifelong gluten-free diet. Again, the biopsy of the small intestine must be done while you're following a gluten-based diet. If you are already following a gluten-free diet when you have your biopsy, it might show a completely normal intestinal lining, or you may have an inconclusive result.

What is the treatment?

Celiac disease is treated with a gluten-free diet, so wheat, barley, rye, and any derived ingredients must all be avoided. The most obvious sources of gluten in the diet are pasta, cereals, breads, flours, pizza bases, pastry, cakes, and cookies. Oats can often be contaminated with other grains, and although most people are able to tolerate uncontaminated oats without a problem, some people with celiac disease may be sensitive and should avoid them. Uncontaminated oats are available, but should be tried under medical advice.

Following a strict gluten-free diet allows the intestines to heal and alleviates symptoms in most cases. Depending on how early the gluten-free diet is started, it can also eliminate the increased risk of osteoporosis and cancer of the small bowel.

What can I eat?

There are plenty of foods that are naturally gluten-free and should be included in your diet. In particular, carbohydrate-rich foods such as potatoes, rice, and corn do not contain gluten. All fresh meat, poultry, and fish, all fresh fruit and vegetables, fresh herbs, individual spices, dried legumes, rice noodles, potatoes, plain nuts, eggs, dairy products, sugar, honey, oils and vinegars, vanilla extract, and fresh and dried yeast are suitable. In fact, the gluten-free diet has the potential to be one of the healthiest diets around because of the increased emphasis placed upon eating fresh, natural, and unprocessed food. If undiagnosed celiac disease has resulted in the poor absorption of vitamins and minerals, a gluten-free diet should soon restore these to healthy levels and lead to a feeling of health and well-being.

More and more manufacturers are producing gluten-free substitute foods, such as gluten-free bread, crackers, and pasta, some of which can be just as good as their gluten-containing equivalents. The Celiac Sprue Association (CSA) publishes a gluten-free book, called *The Celiac's Best Friend*.

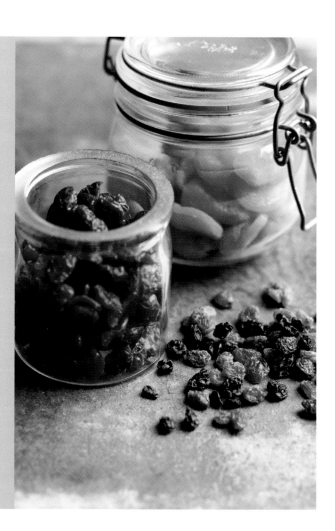

GLUTEN-FREE FOODS

- All fresh meat and fish
- All fresh fruit and vegetables
- Fresh herbs and individual spices
- Cornmeal (polenta)
- Dried legumes, (e.g., peas, lentils, and beans)
- Rice and wild rice
- Rice bran
- Rice noodles
- Plain nuts and seeds
- Eggs
- Dairy products—milk, cream, plain yogurt, cheese
- Soybeans and plain tofu
- Sugar
- Honey
- Corn syrup
- Maple syrup
- Molasses
- Jams and marmalade
- Pure oils and fats
- Vinegars (except malt vinegar)
- Tomato paste
- Vanilla extract
- Fresh and dried yeast

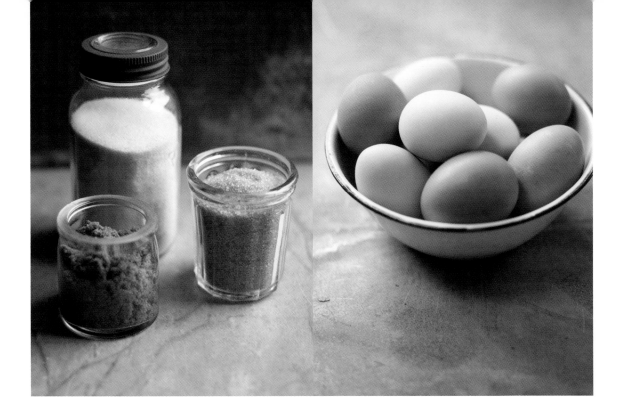

Food labels

Reading labels for hidden sources of gluten from wheat has become much easier thanks to the Food Allergen Labeling and Consumer Protection Act that went into effect in January 2006. It requires the top eight food allergens (which include wheat) to be declared on all product labels. This law also applies to foods that may be imported into the United States.

FOODS AND DRINKS THAT MAY INCLUDE GLUTEN WITHOUT YOU REALIZING IT

- Communion wafers
- Corn tortillas may also contain wheat flour
- Frozen French fries may be coated with flour
- Bouillon cubes and powder
- Vegetable soup may contain pearl barley
- Seasoning mixes
- Mustard products
- Commercial salad dressings and mayonnaise
- Soy sauce (gluten-free brands are available)
- Dry-roasted nuts
- Pretzels

- Bombay mix
- Food that has been deep-fried with other gluten-containing food, e.g., battered fish and chips
- Flavored potato chips
- Some sparkling drinks (alcoholic or non-alcoholic) may contain barley flour to give a cloudy appearance
- Coffee from vending machines
- Malted milk drinks
- Barley water or flavored barley water
- Beer, lager, stout, and ale

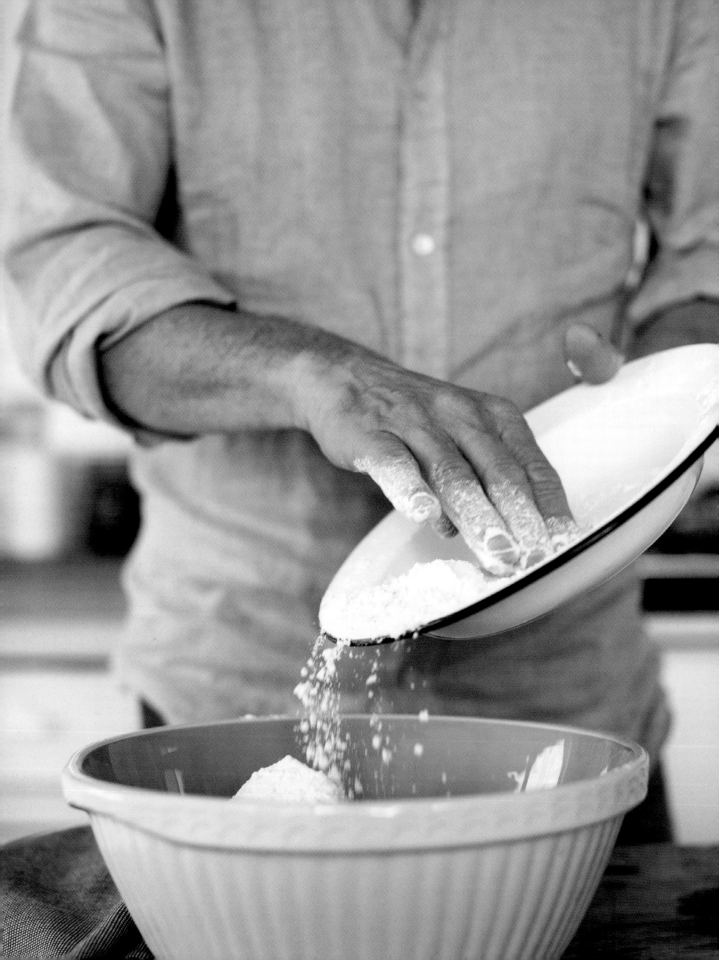

Gluten-free alternatives

In general, it is a good idea to be wary of cereals if you are following a gluten-free diet, but there are a number of naturally gluten-free varieties that are worth knowing about. These give a similar result to cooking with wheat flour and cereals, and will allow you to try recipes that are otherwise out of bounds. As with all other foods, it is best to approach with a degree of caution.

NATURALLY GLUTEN-FREE CEREALS AND GRAINS

- Arrowroot
- Buckwheat flour
- Carob powder
- Chestnut flour
- Cornstarch
- Chickpea flour (Gram flour)
- Flaxseed
- Lotus root powder
- Millet flour
- Cornmeal (polenta)
- Potato flour
- Quinoa flour
- Rice flour
- Sago
- Sorghum flour
- Soy flour
- Tapioca flour
- Teff flour

What about contamination?

Unfortunately, even the tiniest amount of gluten can cause problems for people with celiac disease. Dry gluten-containing ingredients like flour and bread crumbs are high-risk ingredients for contamination and cross-contamination when you are producing gluten-free meals. It is a good idea to keep gluten-free foods separate in the kitchen to make sure you avoid contamination with gluten from other foods.

STEPS TO AVOID CONTAMINATION

- Clean surfaces immediately before use
- Use clean oil for frying potatoes and gluten-free foods (do not reuse oil that has been used for cooking breaded or battered products)
- Keep all pans, utensils, and colanders separate during food preparation and cooking
- Use a clean broiler, separate toaster, or toaster bags to make gluten-free toast
- Make sure that butter, spreads, jellies, pickles, chutneys, and sauces are not contaminated with bread crumbs
- Use squeeze bottles to help avoid contamination through the dipping of spoons or knives

GLUTEN-FREE BAKING—
A CHEF'S PRESCRIPTION

There's no doubt that gluten-free baking is challenging, but with a little practice and the right ingredients, it can also be a lot of fun and extremely satisfying. Some people may even find it difficult to taste the difference between gluten-free recipes and their conventional counterparts!

A few years ago, gluten-free ingredients and products were really few and far between and difficult to get hold of. But thanks to health food stores, some of the supermarkets, and celiac associations such as Celiac Sprue Association (CSA), things are really beginning to change.

An increasing number of food companies are embracing and recognizing the problems that celiac disease poses. There have been major breakthroughs in many products such as cakes, crackers, pasta, cookies, muffins, and bread. Yes, bread! On the ingredients front, gluten-free flour mixes, pancake mixes, and all sorts of baking products are becoming more widely available, making home cooking easier and more accessible.

The gluten in wheat flour gives bread, cakes, and pastry an appealing texture. Gluten holds the gases that are produced when cakes, and particularly breads, rise. So gluten is ordinarily a major factor in giving baked products their characteristic structure. Bread made without gluten is less chewy and lacks the characteristic springy quality, while cakes and pastry can turn out drier and more crumbly. One essential ingredient in gluten-free baking is the exotic-sounding xanthan gum. It acts as a gluten replacement and helps produce great results; turn to page 17 for more about this "magic" ingredient!

Using a blend of gluten-free flours such as rice, potato, and tapioca can replicate wheat flour, and ingredients such as ground almonds are often used in gluten-free baking to help develop flavor and texture. In this book I use three different flour mixes (see page 22), two of which are great for pastries and cakes, so give a lighter finished result. The third flour mix contains soy flour, which means it has a higher protein content. The soy flour mixture can cope better with yeast and helps hold the structure of the finished product, so is ideal for bread.

I have purposely steered clear of using additives that can be bought from specialist companies in these recipes. This is because I prefer not to use them, and I'm sure you probably do too; some are incredibly hard to find, while others are simply just too expensive. Also, I'm not convinced that adding too many chemicals and enhancers is a good thing for the sake of that tiny bit of extra lift or slightly lighter texture.

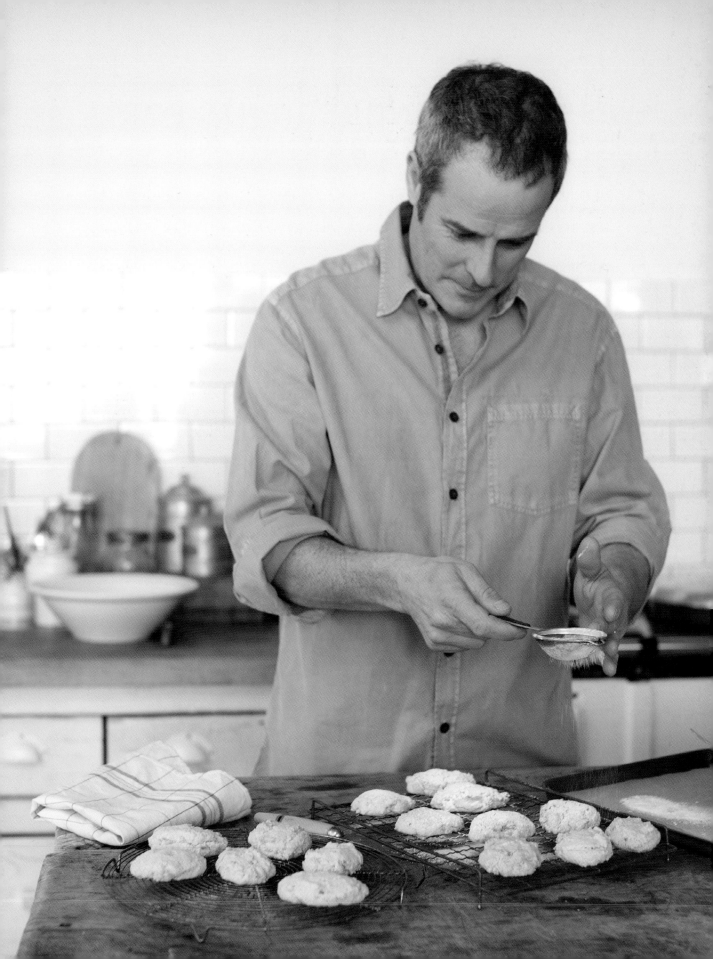

ESSENTIAL INGREDIENTS FOR GLUTEN-FREE BAKING

An ever-increasing variety of gluten-free baking products are available from health food stores and in the "free from" aisle of major supermarkets. Certain gluten-free products help give great results and replicate the quality of conventional baked items. The following are all used in this book; some will be familiar and some are more specialized, but all can really make a difference to the end results of the recipes.

Gluten-free flours

Baking with gluten-free flour and getting successful results can initially seem a challenge, but in fact there is a range of different flours available for the gluten-free cook. These flours can produce crumbly results, but in the Basics chapter I give three recipes for gluten-free flour mixes (see page 22) that give great results. These combinations are used in many of the recipes in the book, so it's worth making a batch of each so they're ready to use when you're in the mood for baking!

These are the flours I use in the mixes:

Brown rice flour is a creamy-colored flour that is easy to digest. It has a slightly nutty flavor and a grainy, rather heavy texture. It is usually combined with other flours for cooking because of its texture.

Chestnut flour has a mildly nutty flavor and is very fine in texture. Chestnut flour is expensive but you can use fine cornmeal in Gluten-Free Flour Mix B as a cheaper alternative.

Cornstarch is used widely as a thickener for sauces. Cornstarch is milled from corn into a fine white powder and has a bland taste, which makes it ideal for baking.

Fine cornmeal (polenta) is an Italian staple made by grinding corn to make a rich yellow flour. It has a slightly sweet flavor and can be used to make cakes, as well as a gluten-free flour mix.

Fine white rice flour is milled from polished white rice. It has a light texture and a bland flavor, so is great for recipes that require a light texture.

Potato flour has a distinctive potato flavor and a heavy texture. It is great for blending with other flours, and a little goes a long way. Do check the date on this flour before blending, as it does not have a very long shelf life. Potato flour should not be confused with potato starch, which is a different product.

Soy flour is made by grinding roasted yellow soybeans. It has a pale yellow color, a nutty taste, and a high protein content. It is best combined with other flours to form an alternative to wheat flour. It is particularly good in breads, as the protein helps to produce a good texture.

Tapioca flour is made from the root of the cassava plant, which is native to the West Indies and South America. When ground, the root forms a soft, sweet, light, fine white flour, making it a good addition to any gluten-free flour mix.

Other useful ingredients

Xanthan gum is produced by fermentation and is a natural type of starch. It improves the texture and shelf life of baked products. When added to gluten-free flour mixes, it replaces the gluten "stretch factor." It works like gluten by binding ingredients during the baking process to give a conventional texture. It can be bought at health food stores and specialist markets, and comes in a powder form that dissolves easily in water. Xanthan gum should be combined with your gluten-free flour mix before adding any liquid.

Glycerin is fabulous for keeping moisture in steamed puddings, cookies, and cakes. It comes in liquid form and you can buy it from pharmacies and chain stores.

Baking powder (see box, page 19) helps to give a light and airy texture to baked products.

Dried yeast I always use quick-rise active dry yeast, normally a ¼-oz packet.

Egg adds great texture and helps hold the gluten-free flour together.

Margarine I've tried a variety of different types and have found Land O'Lakes and Fleischmann's margarine will both work well.

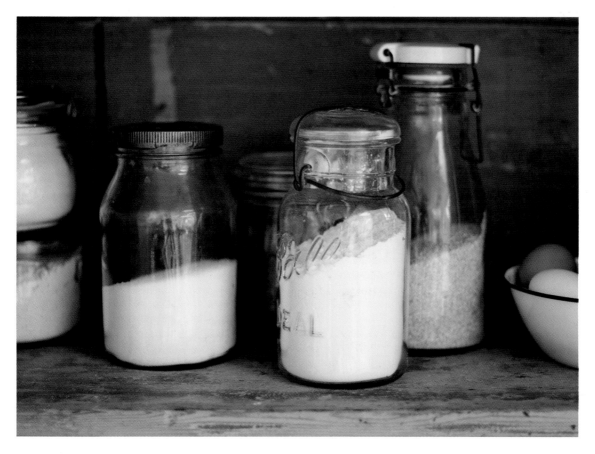

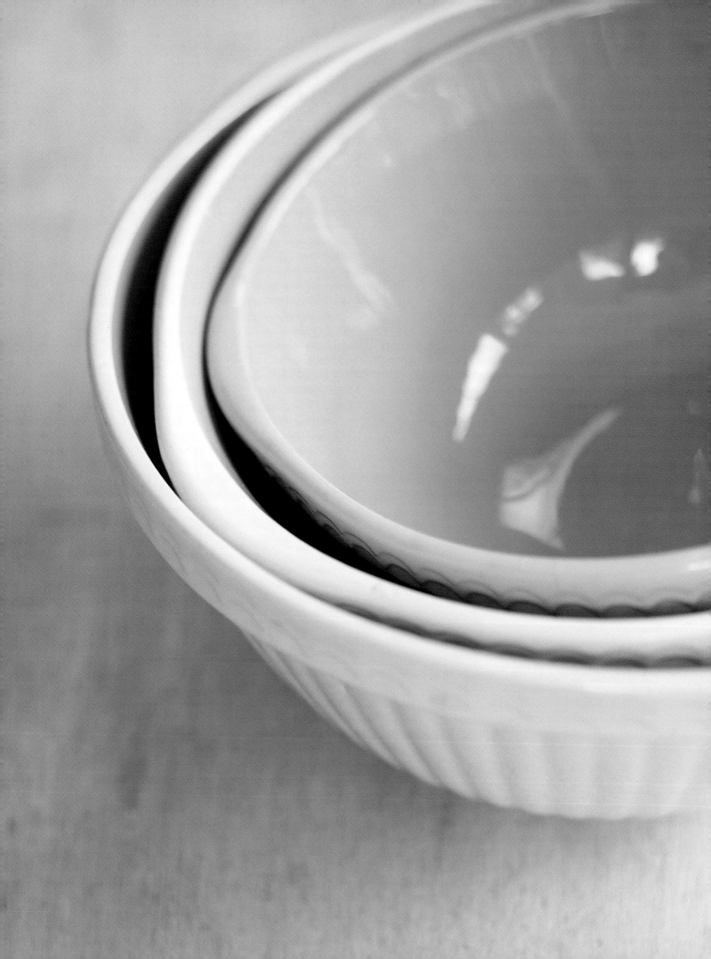

NOTES ON THE RECIPES

Here are a few things to consider before you start baking!

Gluten-free ingredients to check before use

Several ingredients are, strictly speaking, gluten-free, provided they come from a source where there is no risk of contamination. They are used in recipes in this book, but please always check the label before use. You can also check the book *The Celiac's Best Friend* published by the Celiac Sprue Association (CSA). See contact details on page 170.

CHECK THE CELIAC SPRUE ASSOCIATION'S BOOK, *THE CELIAC'S BEST FRIEND* FOR SUITABLE PRODUCTS OF THE FOLLOWING:

- Baking powder
- Chocolate—milk, white and bittersweet
- Cake decorations, e.g., chocolate sprinkles, edible glitter
- Oats
- Marshmallows
- Custard—ready-made and powder
- Marzipan
- Meringues
- Shortbread
- Fine cornmeal
- Crisp puffed rice cereal
- Cream cheese

Cooking notes

- All teaspoon and tablespoon measurements are level
- A 750W microwave was used throughout
- If you are using a convection oven, please refer to the manufacturer's handbook for the correct oven temperature conversion

How long do the products last?

Many of the cakes, cookies, and breads in the book can be frozen, and each recipe has freezing instructions, along with storage instructions. An extra tip I've got to share is that warming gluten-free products, including cookies, in a microwave for a few seconds, or gently in a warm oven for a very short time, makes them soft and pliable again.

And for the very best results ...

Finally, after lots of testing, testing, and testing again, I have found that it's critical that the recipes are adhered to exactly when measuring out all the ingredients, following the method, and using the cooking instructions.

   I know you will be as delighted with the results of these recipes as I have been—so now it's time to get into the kitchen, start cooking, and enjoy!

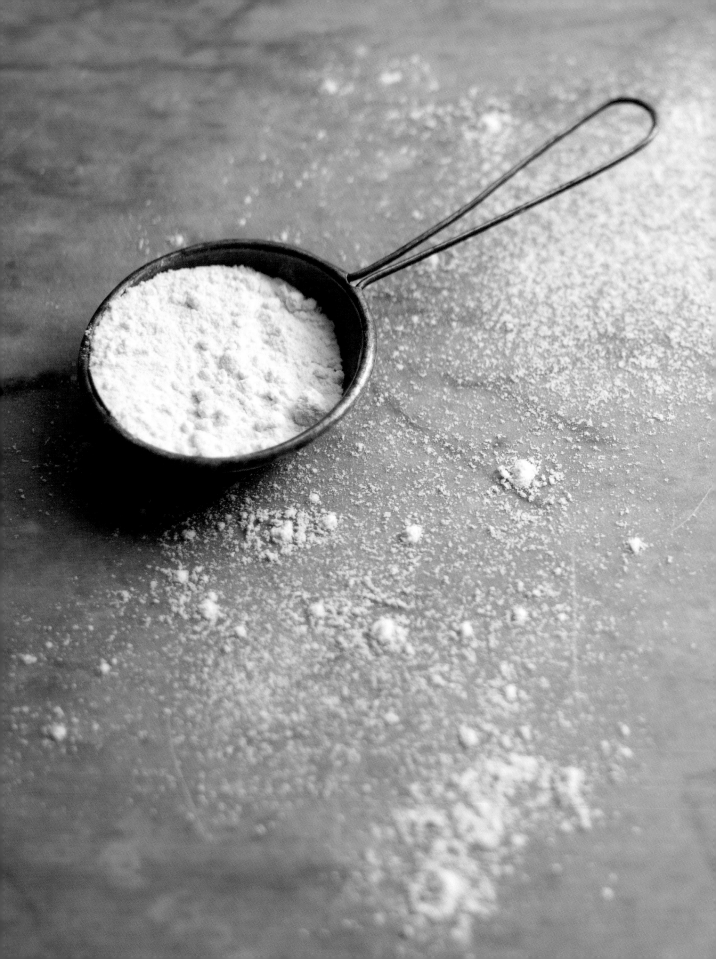

BASICS

GLUTEN-FREE FLOUR MIXES

I use three Gluten-Free Flour Mixes in this book, simply because different combinations of flour work better for different recipes. Gluten-Free Flour Mixes A and B work well for cookies and cakes, while the Gluten-Free Bread Mix contains soy flour, which has a high protein content and helps most of the recipes with yeast. Make sure you check the "best before" date of all the flours you are using, make a note of the earliest date and use the flour before then.

GLUTEN-FREE FLOUR MIX A

MAKES: 7¼ CUPS (2¼ LB)
PREPARATION: 5 MINUTES

5¼ cups (25 oz) fine white rice flour

1 cup (7 oz) potato flour

1 cup (3½ oz) tapioca flour

Mix all the flours together very thoroughly, or put into a food processor and pulse until mixed. Store in an airtight container.

GLUTEN-FREE BREAD MIX

MAKES: APPROX. 10¾ CUPS (2¾ LB)
PREPARATION: 5 MINUTES

4½ cups (14 oz) soy flour

2 cups (7 oz) tapioca flour

2 cups (14 oz) potato flour

2¼ cups (10½ oz) cornstarch

Mix all the flours together very thoroughly, or put into a food processor and pulse until mixed. Store in an airtight container.

GLUTEN-FREE FLOUR MIX B

MAKES: 8¼ CUPS (2¼ LB)
PREPARATION: 5 MINUTES

2½ cups (10½ oz) fine cornmeal
   (see box, page 19) or chestnut
   flour

4¼ cups (18 oz) brown rice flour

1½ cups (7 oz) cornstarch

Mix all the flours together very thoroughly, or put into a food processor and pulse until mixed. Store in an airtight container.

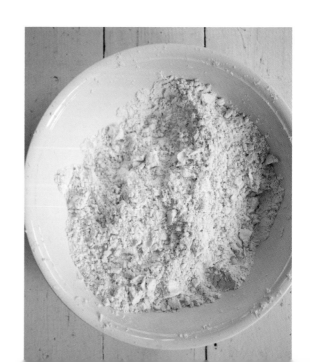

SHORTBREAD

This recipe works well as a base for a bar cookie or sheet cake, but it can also be turned into tasty cookies to nibble with a cup of tea.

MAKES: ONE 9-INCH (23 CM) SQUARE SHORTBREAD BASE OR APPROXIMATELY 12–14 COOKIES

PREPARATION: 10 MINUTES

BAKING: 15–20 MINUTES

¾ cup (3½ oz) cornstarch

¾ cup (3½ oz) rice flour

¼ cup (2 oz) superfine sugar

2 tablespoons soft light brown sugar

½ cup (4 oz) unsalted butter, cubed

cornstarch, for dusting

light brown or superfine sugar, for sprinkling on cookies

Preheat the oven to 375°F (190°C).

Put the flours and sugars into a food processor and blend together. Add the butter and pulse until the mixture starts to clump together.

For a shortbread base: Line a 9-inch (23 cm) square pan with parchment paper. Tip the crumb mixture into the pan, and press very lightly to make an even layer. Bake the base in the oven for about 15 minutes, or until pale golden brown.

For shortbread cookies: Press the crumbs lightly into a dough, and roll out thickly on a cornstarch-dusted board. Press or cut into shape, transfer to a nonstick baking sheet or a baking sheet lined with parchment paper, and bake for 12–14 minutes. Allow to cool on the sheet, and sprinkle with light brown or superfine sugar, to serve.

☐ **TO STORE:** The base and cookies will keep for up to 1 week in an airtight container.

✱ **TO FREEZE:** Wrap well, and freeze in an airtight container. Defrost to room temperature before using.

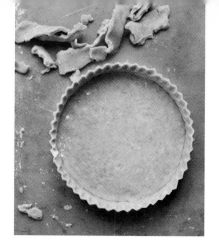

SHORT PASTRY

In *Seriously Good! Gluten-Free Cooking* I gave a recipe for pastry. Here is another version, but this time I have added a teaspoon of xanthan gum, an egg, and slightly more water, which really makes a big difference to the end result. If you don't have xanthan gum, you can substitute two teaspoons of psyllium husk (both are available from health food stores), but if using the latter, you will need to add a little more water, as the absorption rate is higher.

MAKES: ONE 1½-INCH (4 CM) DEEP, 9½-INCH (24 CM) ROUND TART CRUST
PREPARATION: 10 MINUTES
BAKING: 15–20 MINUTES

2¼ cups (8 oz) Gluten-Free Flour Mix A (see page 22)

1 teaspoon xanthan gum

2 pinches of salt

½ cup (4 oz) margarine

1 large egg, beaten, at room temperature

Place the flour, xanthan gum, and salt in a mixing bowl, and mix really well. Add the margarine, and rub in until you have achieved the consistency of fine bread crumbs. I tend to take the lazy route and use a food processor. Add the egg and a little water, and mix really well. Keep an eye on the texture—you may need to add a little more water so it is nice and soft; bear in mind the xanthan gum will tighten up the mixture considerably. Roll out and use as required.

To make a tart crust: Roll out the pastry, to a circle approximately 12 inches (30 cm) in diameter, on a cornstarch-dusted work surface. Transfer to a 1½-inch (4 cm) deep, 9½-inch (24 cm) pan, and line with parchment paper and dried beans.

Bake for 10 minutes at 350°F (180°C), then reduce the temperature to 325°F (160°C) for 10–15 minutes.

Lift out the parchment paper and beans carefully, brush thickly with beaten egg, covering any cracks, and return to the oven for 5–6 minutes to just set the egg. Brush with egg again, and bake for another 5 minutes.

☐ **TO STORE:** Wrap the dough in plastic wrap, and refrigerate for up to 2 days.

✳ **TO FREEZE:** Not suitable.

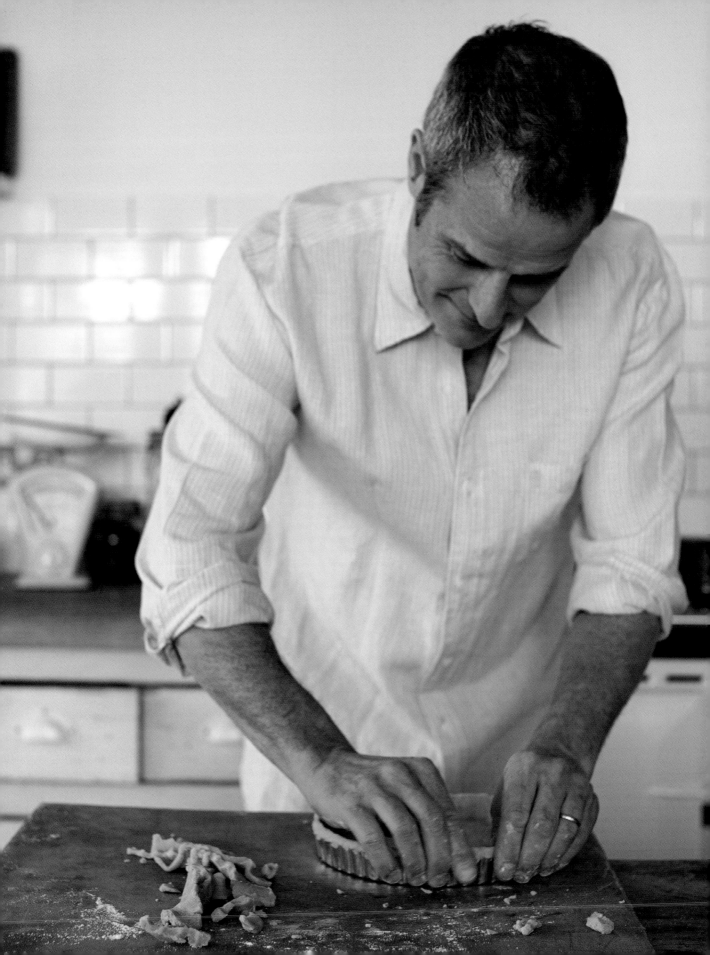

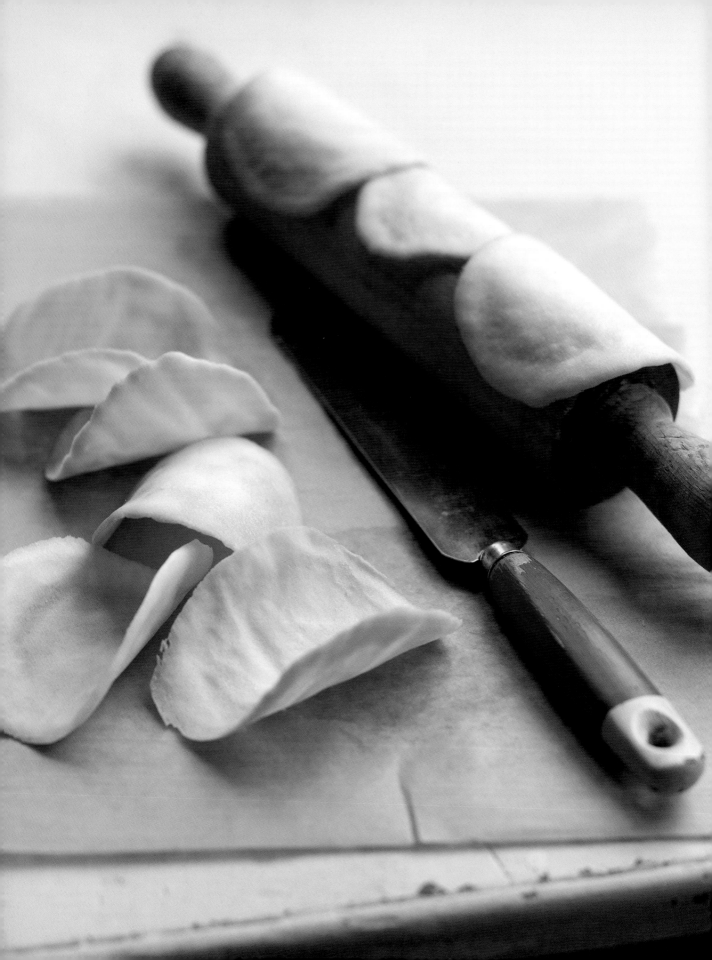

TUILES

This is the classic cookie chefs serve with ice creams and sorbets. They are very easy to make and look quite professional. The two-stage cooking process ensures a nice even color to the cookie.

These can be baked and pressed over the bottom of an upturned teacup or mug to make decorative cases to hold mousses, ice creams, and sorbets. The unbaked mixture will keep, covered, in the fridge for a couple of weeks.

MAKES: ABOUT 12–14 COOKIES
PREPARATION: 10 MINUTES
BAKING: 15 MINUTES

---

2 medium egg whites, at room temperature

¾ cup (3½ oz) confectioners' sugar, sifted

generous ½ cup (3 oz) Gluten-Free Flour Mix A (see page 22)

6 tablespoons (3 oz) unsalted butter, melted

Place the egg whites, confectioners' sugar, and flour into a bowl and beat together. Add the warm melted butter, and again beat well. Chill in the fridge for at least 2 hours.

When you are ready to bake the cookies, preheat the oven to 350°F (180°C). Line a baking sheet with parchment paper (you will need to cook these in batches).

Spoon out about a teaspoon-sized blob of the mixture onto the sheet, and spread it out as thinly as possible with a palette knife; you may only get 2–3 to a sheet, as the mixture will expand. Bake until the cookies are just set but have no color—this is called poaching.

Remove the sheet from the oven, and leave the cookies to cool for about 5 minutes. Then bake the cookies for 2–3 minutes more until they are a nice golden color.

Remove the sheet from the oven, and using a palette knife, quickly and carefully lift off the cookies and lay them over a rolling pin, placed on a kitchen towel to stop it moving, to cool. You have to be quick at this point, or the cookies will set and crack very quickly. The size is up to you—I think the bigger the better!

☐ **TO STORE:** Carefully transfer the cooled cookies to an airtight container for up to 1 week, taking care as they are quite fragile.

✱ **TO FREEZE:** Not suitable.

VANILLA CUPCAKES

Cupcakes are all the rage at the moment, and they come in many different shapes and sizes, from baby cakes to giant versions that you can fill with ice cream.

The good thing, though, is that you don't need to be a baker or experienced cook to make them! This recipe has four simple steps, and hey presto, they're ready to pop into the oven. So add what you like to this basic recipe, and have a bit of fun. I think this recipe is softer and tastier than a standard sponge cake recipe.

MAKES: 12 CUPCAKES
PREPARATION: 15 MINUTES
BAKING: 15–20 MINUTES

---

generous ¾ cup (6½ oz) superfine sugar

2 large eggs, at room temperature

1 teaspoon vanilla extract

1 teaspoon glycerin

generous 1¼ cups (7 oz) Gluten-Free Flour Mix A (see page 22)

1½ teaspoons baking powder (see box, page 19)

½ teaspoon xanthan gum

½ cup (4 fl oz) + 2 teaspoons sunflower oil

½ cup (4 fl oz) + 2 teaspoons whole milk

Preheat the oven to 350°F (180°C). Place 12 paper muffin cup liners in a muffin pan.

Place the superfine sugar, eggs, vanilla, and glycerin into a large mixing bowl, and beat with a hand-held electric mixer on high speed for 4 minutes.

Meanwhile, combine the flour, baking powder, and xanthan gum together, and mix them really well. I find it best to sift them a couple of times, to make sure the ingredients are fully incorporated.

Next, mix the oil and milk together in a measuring cup.

Once the egg mixture is nice and thick, add the flour mixture and liquid. Beat well, but don't go mad.

Divide the mixture between the muffin cups. Bake for 15–20 minutes, or until well risen to the top of the paper liners. Remove the cupcakes in the liners from the pan, and allow to cool on a wire rack.

Ice and decorate however you like.

Try a different flavor ...
Add any of the following to the egg mixture with the flour: ⅓ cup (2 oz) dried fruit, ½ cup (3 oz) fresh berries, ⅓ cup (2 oz) chopped bittersweet chocolate, ½ cup (2 oz) chopped nuts, zest of 1 lemon or 1 orange.

☐ **TO STORE:** Store in an airtight container for up to 1 week.

✳ **TO FREEZE:** Once cooled, store either in a plastic bag or an airtight container.

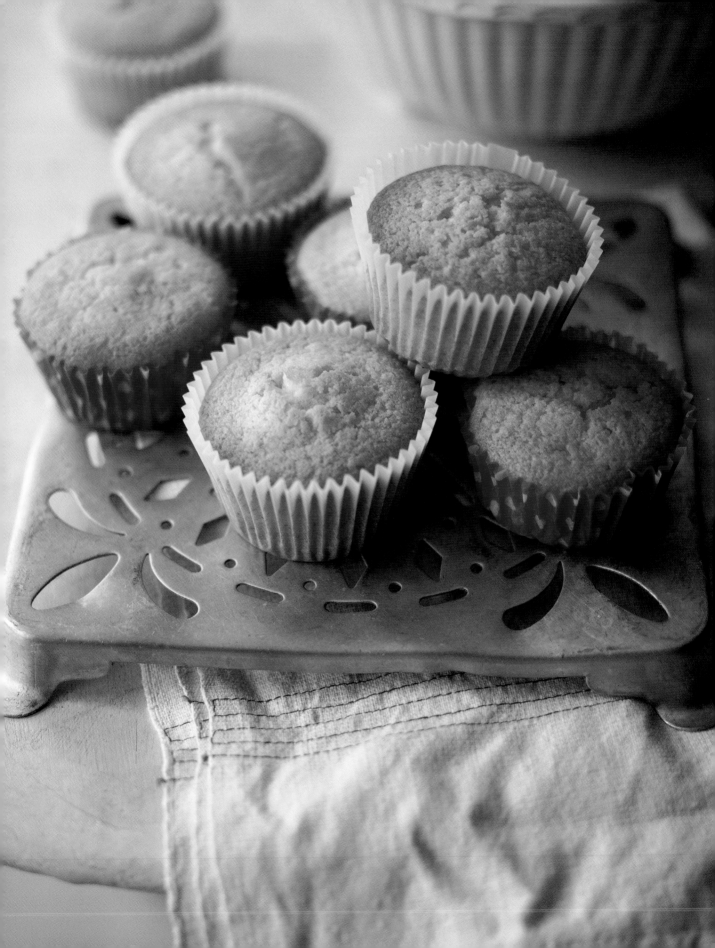

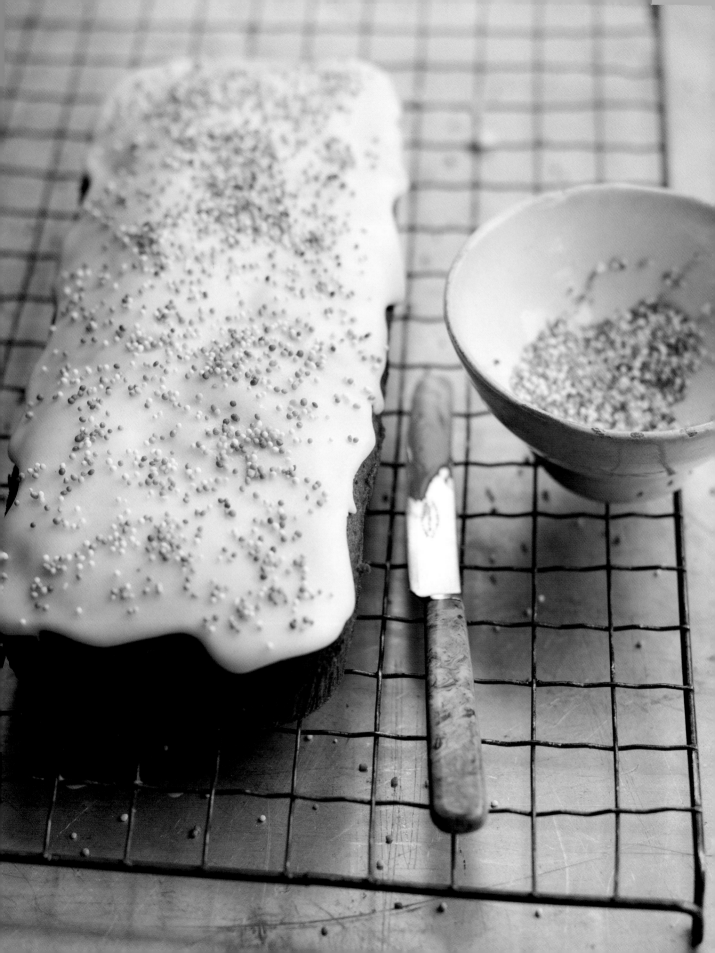

LIGHT SPONGE CAKE

This is a variation on a basic sponge cake recipe. It can be served whole, drizzled with your favorite frosting, or cut into individual pieces and frosted and decorated with candy, chocolate chips, edible glitter ... the choices are endless!

Making sure the margarine and eggs are at room temperature and the milk is warmed with the glycerin will ensure the maximum lift from the sponge when baking. The addition of glycerin helps retain moisture in the cake's structure. I use disposable foil trays to bake this cake, then carefully wash them and use again.

MAKES: ONE 9 × 5-INCH
(23 × 13 CM, 2 LB) LOAF
PREPARATION: 15 MINUTES
BAKING: 20–30 MINUTES

---

vegetable oil, for oiling

1¼ generous cups (7 oz) Gluten-Free Flour Mix A (see page 22)

1 teaspoon baking soda

1 teaspoon baking powder (see box, page 19)

6 tablespoons (3 oz) margarine

⅔ cup (5 oz) superfine sugar

2 large eggs, at room temperature

generous ½ cup (4 fl oz) 2% milk, warmed with 1 teaspoon glycerin

Preheat the oven to 325°F (160°C). Lightly oil a 9 × 5-inch (23 × 13 cm, 2 lb) loaf pan.

Place the flour, baking soda, and baking powder into a bowl and mix well.

Warm a large mixing bowl under hot running water. Place the margarine and sugar in the bowl, and beat until light and creamy (warming the bowl makes it easier to cream the margarine and sugar together).

Add the flour mixture to the margarine and sugar, along with the eggs, and mix well. Add the warm milk and glycerin, and mix to a batter consistency, then spoon or pour into the prepared pan.

Bake for 20–25 minutes, or until risen and lightly colored. Remove and cool on a wire rack.

Ice and decorate however you like.

☐ **TO STORE:** Store in an airtight container for 2–3 days.

✳ **TO FREEZE:** Either freeze the uniced cake whole or cut into slices and wrap well in plastic wrap.

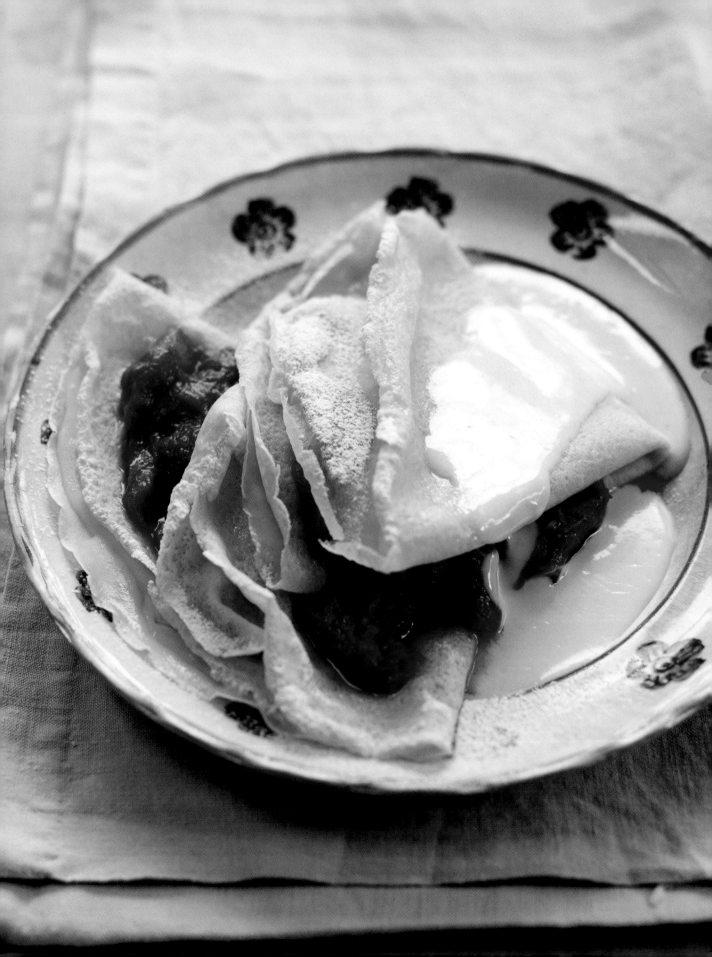

CLASSIC CRÊPES

Everyone likes a crêpe and I have had many requests for a gluten-free version. So here is a good basic recipe that I first cooked on the TV show *This Morning*.

MAKES: 4–6 CRÊPES
PREPARATION: 15 MINUTES
COOKING: 6–8 MINUTES

---

generous ¾ cup (3¼ oz) brown
    rice flour

¼ cup (1¼ oz) cornstarch

pinch of salt

2 large eggs, at room
    temperature

approximately 1 scant cup
    (7 fl oz) 2% milk

3 tablespoons vegetable oil

To make the crêpes, stir the brown rice flour, cornstarch, and salt together in a medium mixing bowl. Add the eggs and three-quarters of the milk, and whisk well until thoroughly combined. The mixture should be a similar consistency to thick heavy cream; add more milk if necessary.

Heat the vegetable oil in a 9-inch nonstick skillet over medium heat. Add 4 tablespoons of batter to the pan and swirl it around to coat the base. Cook for 30–60 seconds, then start to loosen the edges of the crêpe with an offset spatula. Once the crêpe is set, turn it over, using the offset spatula (or you can flip it in the air if you're feeling brave!), and cook the second side for 30–60 seconds, or until golden brown. Repeat until all the batter is used up. Stack the crêpes on a plate and cover them with foil to keep them warm.

Serve with your preferred topping (see mine below)!

RHUBARB & CUSTARD CRÊPES

approximately 1 heaping cup
    (8 oz) rhubarb, cut into
    ¾-inch (2cm) pieces
finely grated zest and juice
    of 1 large lemon

1 vanilla bean, split

4 tablespoons superfine sugar,
    plus extra, to taste

2 cups (8 oz) ready-made
    custard (see box, page 19)

4–6 crêpes (see above)

Place the rhubarb in a medium pan. Add the lemon zest and juice, vanilla bean, and sugar, and cook over low heat for about 15 minutes, stirring occasionally; the rhubarb will break down nicely. Keep warm.

Warm the custard following the package instructions. Warm the crêpes in the microwave for 10 seconds each.

To serve, lay a warm crêpe on a plate, spoon on some rhubarb, fold over, and spoon on a little custard. You could add a little ice cream or a blob of whipped cream if you really wanted to make it extra special.

☐ **TO STORE:** The plain crêpes can be stacked, wrapped in plastic wrap, and stored in the fridge for 3–4 days.

✳ **TO FREEZE:** Not suitable.

BUTTERMILK PANCAKES

I really like these pancakes—they are great for breakfast or a late brunch. I find, once cooked, it is best to keep them warm in a clean kitchen towel, then reheat them before eating (10 seconds in the microwave per pancake is plenty).

MAKES: 8–10 PANCAKES
PREPARATION: 15 MINUTES
COOKING: 25 MINUTES

---

1 scant cup (4 oz) fine rice flour

½ teaspoon baking powder
(see box, page 19)

pinch of salt

1 large egg, at room
temperature

1½ tablespoons sunflower oil

4 tablespoons (2 oz) unsalted
butter, melted

1¼ cups (10 fl oz) buttermilk

3 tablespoons mild olive oil

To make the pancakes, place the rice flour, baking powder, and salt in a medium mixing bowl. Place the egg, sunflower oil, melted butter, and buttermilk in a bowl and whisk well together. Gradually add the wet mixture to the dry ingredients, stirring well between each addition; you should end up with a loose but thickish batter.

Heat a 9-inch (23 cm) nonstick skillet over medium heat and add the olive oil.

Spoon in 4 separate tablespoons of batter to make 4 small pancakes. Cook for 2–3 minutes on one side, then flip over and cook the other side until it is light brown. Repeat until all the batter is used up. Stack the pancakes on a plate, and cover them with foil to keep them warm.

Topping ideas
- Maple syrup and blueberries
- Corn syrup and whipped cream
- Crème fraîche and brown sugar
- Crushed bananas and peanut butter

☐ **TO STORE:** The plain pancakes can be stacked, wrapped in plastic wrap, and stored in the fridge for 2 days.

✳ **TO FREEZE:** Not suitable.

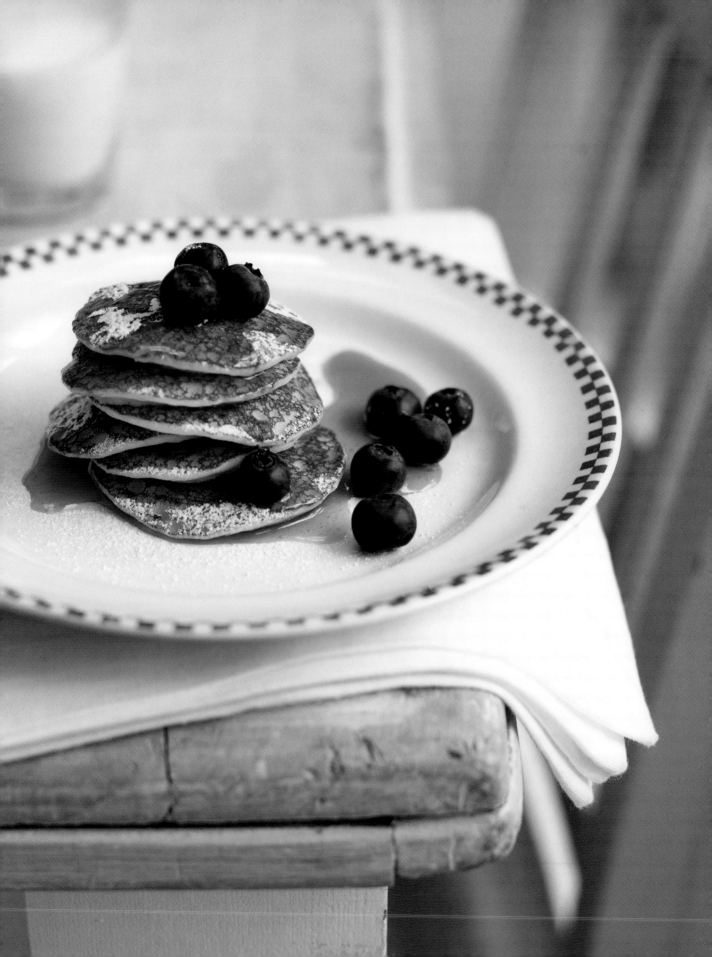

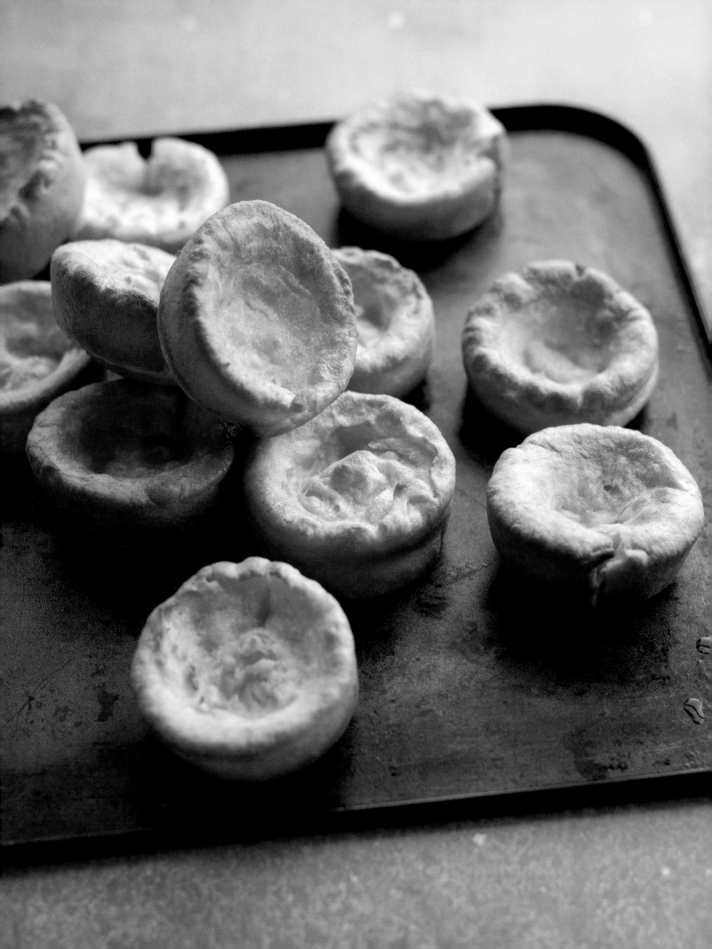

YORKSHIRE PUDDINGS (POPOVERS)

I often use a muffin pan to make Yorkshire puddings because it is slightly deeper, helping to give the puddings more structure when baked. I have also found that baking these in a black nonstick popover pan makes them rise higher than when they're baked in an plain pan.

MAKES: 10–12 PUDDINGS
PREPARATION: 15 MINUTES
BAKING: 20–25 MINUTES

10–12 tablespoons olive oil

1 generous cup (5½ oz) Gluten-Free Flour Mix A (see page 22)

1 generous cup (5 oz) cornstarch

4 large eggs, at room temperature

1¼ cups (10 fl oz) 2% milk

salt and freshly ground black pepper

Preheat the oven to 425°F (220°C).

Place a tablespoon of olive oil into each cup of a 10–12 cup muffin pan or popover pan. Place the pan on a baking sheet, and put it into the oven for 10 minutes to heat up.

Meanwhile, place the flour and cornstarch in a deep mixing bowl. Add the eggs and milk, and whisk until well blended. Add a little salt and pepper. Pour into the oiled pans so that they are just over half full, and return to the oven. Bake for 20–25 minutes, or until well risen and nicely browned. Serve immediately.

☐ **TO STORE:** Not suitable.

✳ **TO FREEZE:** Freeze the Yorkshire puddings once thoroughly cooled. Flash through a hot oven to crisp up.

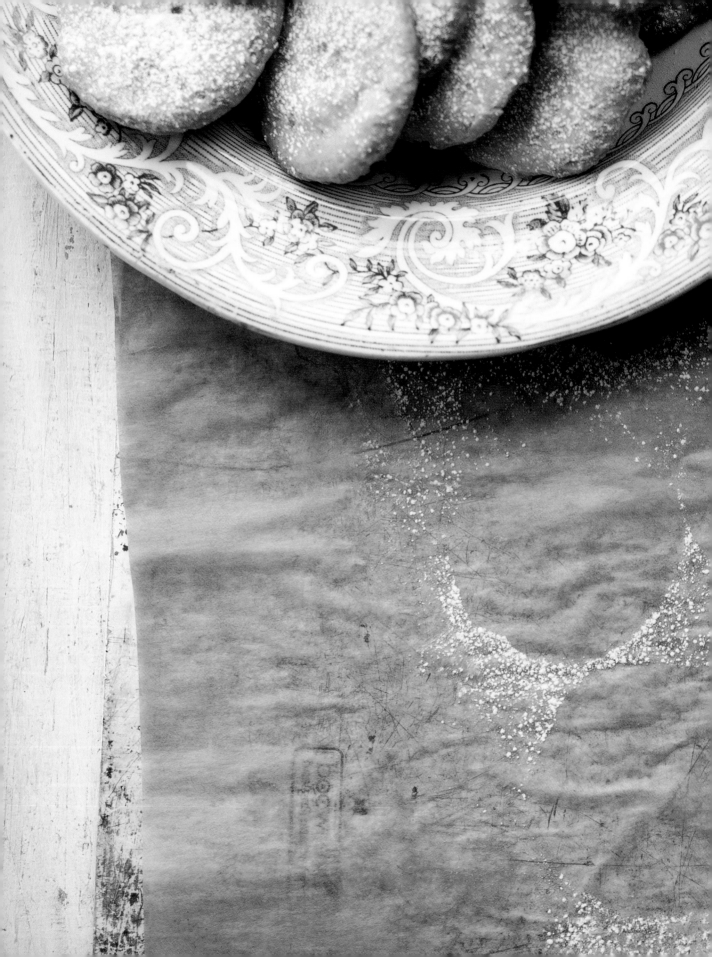

COOKIES

SOFT ZESTY LEMON FONDANT COOKIES

The zestiness of these cookies does it for me, and making up the topping using fondant icing sugar with lemon juice gives the icing a really acidic kick. Fondant icing sugar is confectioners' sugar with glucose added, so it sets at room temperature with a lovely shine, similar to the eclairs you can buy at bakeries. Make it by adding 1 teaspoon light corn syrup to 1 cup (4 oz) confectioners' sugar as below.

MAKES: 12 COOKIES
PREPARATION: 15 MINUTES
BAKING: 15–20 MINUTES

1½ cups (7 oz) Gluten-Free Flour
  Mix A (see page 22)

6 tablespoons (3 oz) margarine

¼ teaspoon baking powder
  (see box, page 19)

pinch of salt

6 tablespoons superfine sugar

1 large egg, at room
  temperature

1 teaspoon glycerin

zest and juice of 1 large lemon

½ cup (2 oz) confectioners'
  sugar

½ teaspoon light corn syrup

extra lemon zest, to decorate

Place the flour, margarine, baking powder, salt, and sugar in a food processor, and blitz until you have achieved the consistency of fine bread crumbs. Add the egg, glycerin, and lemon zest, and mix. Lightly bring together on a floured surface, and then form into a 6–8-inch (15–20 cm) cylinder. Wrap in plastic wrap and chill well.

Preheat the oven to 400°F (200°C). Line two baking sheets with parchment paper (you will need to bake these in batches).

When you are ready to bake the cookies, cut off ¼-inch (5 mm) slices of the dough, and place them on the lined sheets. Bake for 15–20 minutes, or until baked and lightly browned. Then transfer to a wire rack to cool.

Meanwhile, place the lemon juice in a small bowl, then add the confectioners' sugar and corn syrup, and beat until smooth. You may need to adjust the consistency with a little water (softer) or extra confectioners' sugar (firmer). Coat the cookies thickly with the frosting, decorate with lemon zest, and leave to set.

☐ **TO STORE:** Store the cooled cookies in an airtight container for up to 1 week.

✱ **TO FREEZE:** The dough and the baked unfrosted cookies freeze well.
For the dough: Wrap it in plastic wrap, and freeze. Defrost for 1 hour, or until soft enough to cut and bake as above.
For the cookies: Wrap well, and store in an airtight container. Defrost for 30 minutes, then heat through at 350°F (180°C) for 2–3 minutes to soften again. Frost once cooled.

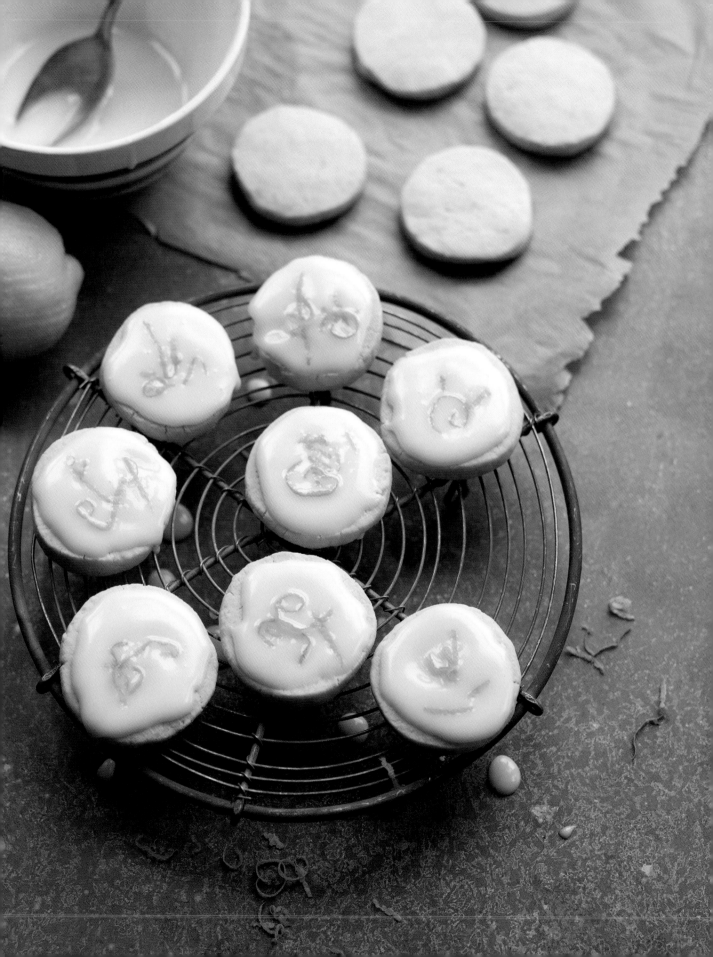

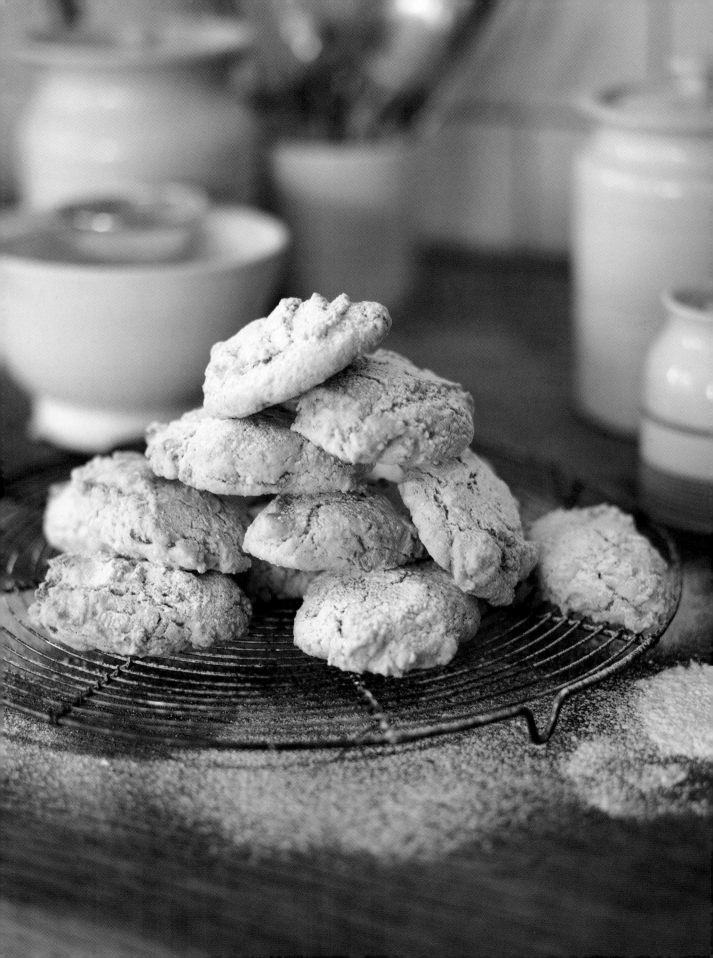

SOFT PINE NUT COOKIES

I spent a few years working in northern Italy, and every couple of weeks we would go to a pesto factory in Asti where I was helping develop recipes. We would pass a very small bakery on the way to the factory in the mornings. In the window they had many breads and cakes, but in one corner there were small meringue cookies, which were delicious. Here is my version, light and packed full of flavor.

MAKES: ABOUT 20 COOKIES
PREPARATION: 15 MINUTES
BAKING: 30 MINUTES

1¾ cups (7 oz) slivered
   almonds

1 scant cup (3½ oz) pine nuts

¾ cup (3½ oz) rice flour

1 cup (8 oz) superfine sugar

zest of 1 lemon

2 large egg whites,
   at room temperature

pinch of cream of tartar

½ teaspoon vanilla extract

½ teaspoon almond extract

cinnamon and sifted
   confectioners' sugar,
   for dusting

Preheat the oven to 350°F (180°C). Line a baking sheet with parchment paper.

Place the almonds and pine nuts on the lined sheet, and brown them well in the oven for 8–10 minutes; the almonds will brown slightly quicker. Once browned, remove from the oven and cool. Reduce the oven temperature to 325°F (160°C).

Once cooled, place the almonds and rice flour in a food processor, and blitz until you have a fine mix. Place in a medium mixing bowl, add the pine nuts, ½ cup (4 oz) of the sugar, and the lemon zest, and mix well.

Whisk the egg whites with the cream of tartar until light and foamy, then add the remaining superfine sugar and whisk until creamy and glossy, but do not overbeat. Fold the nut mixture into the egg whites, along with the vanilla and almond extracts.

With a wet teaspoon, drop the mixture into small oval mounds, and place on the lined sheet (you will need to bake these in batches). Flatten each mound slightly before baking. Bake for 15–20 minutes, until they turn light golden, keeping an eye on them, as they brown quickly. Remove and transfer to a wire rack to cool.

Sprinkle with cinnamon and confectioners' sugar.

☐ **TO STORE:** Store the cooled cookies in an airtight container for up to 1 week.

✱ **TO FREEZE:** Freeze the cooled cookies before dusting with the sugar and cinnamon—wrap well, and store in an airtight container. Defrost for 30 minutes, then heat through at 350°F (180°C) for 2–3 minutes to soften again and dust with the sugar and cinnamon.

CHOCOLATE, PEANUT BUTTER & FUDGE COOKIES

This recipe is so simple it's unbelievable—just mix together well and bake! It also has the bonus of using no flour at all. If you slightly underbake the cookies, you will end up with a softer, chewier texture, but if you prefer your cookies slightly crunchier, bake a little longer.

MAKES: 12–14 SOFT COOKIES
PREPARATION: 10 MINUTES
BAKING: 12–14 MINUTES

---

1 large egg, at room temperature

6 tablespoons superfine sugar

½ cup (4½ oz) crunchy peanut butter, at room temperature

pinch or two of chili powder

3 small squares (1½ oz) fudge, finely chopped

¼ cup (1½ oz) bittersweet chocolate (see box, page 19), finely chopped

Preheat the oven to 350°F (180°C). Line two baking sheets with parchment paper (you will need to bake these in batches).

Place the egg and sugar in a bowl, and beat with a whisk. Add the peanut butter and chili powder, and mix well. Add the chopped fudge and chocolate, and mix in.

Spoon tablespoonfuls of the mixture onto the lined baking sheets, and flatten slightly, as the mixture will not spread much, then bake for 12–14 minutes.

When baked, remove the cookies from the paper with an offset spatula, and cool on a wire rack.

☐ **TO STORE:** Store the cooled cookies in an airtight container for up to 1 week.

✳ **TO FREEZE:** The baked, cooled cookies freeze well. Wrap well, and store in an airtight container. Defrost for 30 minutes, then heat through at 350°F (180°C) for 2–3 minutes to soften again.

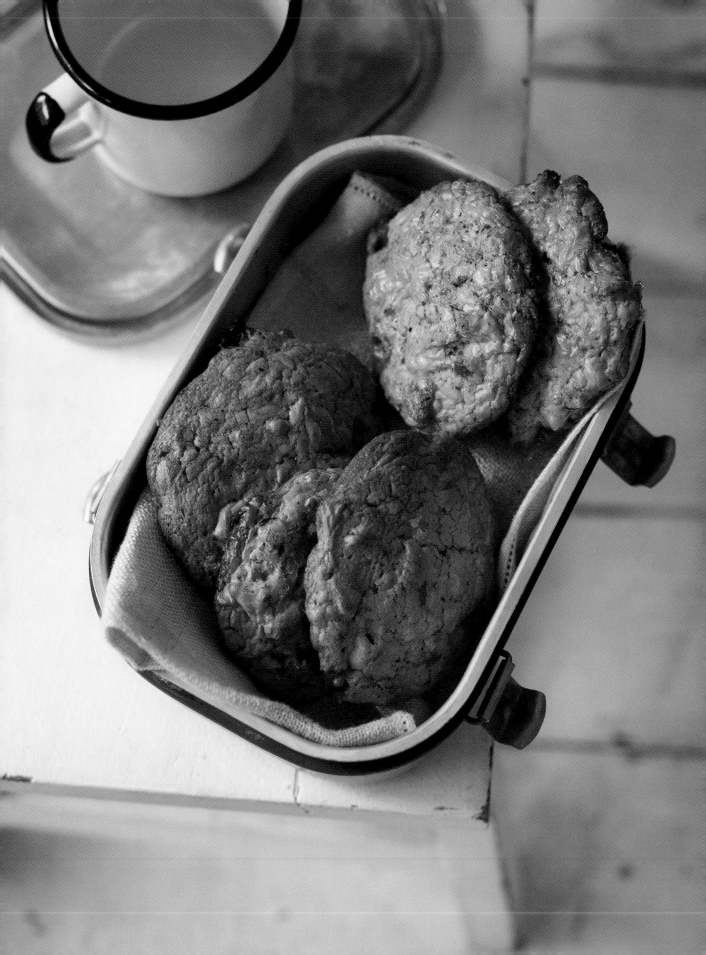

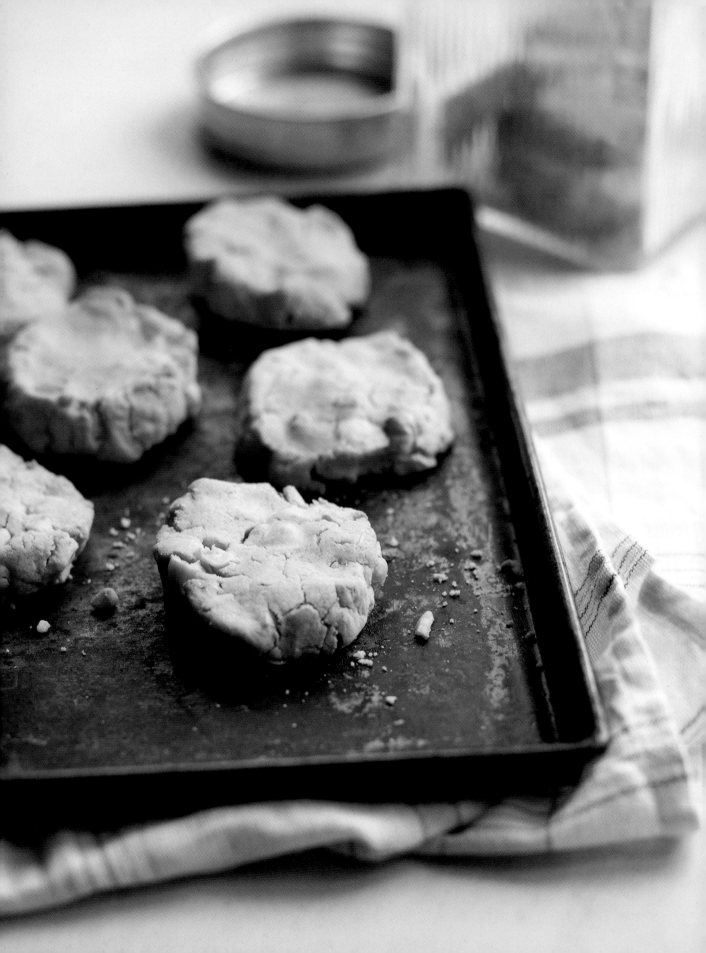

ROASTED HAZELNUT COOKIES

I love roasted hazelnuts; they make a very special cookie or shortbread, and they are widely available in supermarkets. Any nut can be used instead here, but remember to roast them in the oven for an even color (see method for roasting nuts in Soft Pine Nut Cookies, page 43).

MAKES: ABOUT 20 COOKIES
PREPARATION: 15 MINUTES
BAKING: ABOUT 10 MINUTES

---

1 scant cup (4 oz) rice flour

½ cup (2½ oz) cornstarch

½ teaspoon baking powder (see box, page 19)

½ teaspoon ground nutmeg

½ teaspoon pumpkin pie spice

2 tablespoons (1 oz) margarine, softened

3 tablespoons superfine sugar

1 tablespoon light corn syrup

¾ cup (3 oz) roasted hazelnuts, roughly chopped

Preheat the oven to 350°F (180°C). Line two baking sheets with parchment paper (you will need to bake these in batches).

In a medium mixing bowl, combine the flour, cornstarch, baking powder, nutmeg, and pumpkin pie spice, and mix together well. Add the softened margarine, sugar, syrup, and hazelnuts, and mix well.

Spoon the mixture onto the lined baking sheets, using a tablespoon to form 1-inch (2.5 cm) circles. Flatten with a wet finger, then bake for 10 minutes, or until lightly browned.

Once baked, allow the cookies to cool slightly on the sheets, then transfer to a wire rack to cool completely.

☐ **TO STORE:** Store the cooled cookies in an airtight container for up to 1 week.

✳ **TO FREEZE:** The raw dough freezes well. Wrap it in plastic wrap, and freeze. Defrost for 1 hour, or until soft enough to cut and bake as above.

JEWELED FLORENTINES

Delicious little treats of toasted nuts and candied fruits, caramelized into lacy cookies and half coated in milk chocolate. Florentines make a great gift at any time, or just enjoy them with a shot of espresso.

MAKES: ABOUT 12–14 COOKIES
PREPARATION: 20 MINUTES
BAKING: 10 MINUTES

---

2 tablespoons (1 oz) unsalted butter

⅓ cup (2½ oz) superfine sugar

2 teaspoons clear honey

1 tablespoon rice flour

2½ tablespoons mixed candied peel, chopped

¼ cup (2 oz) candied cherries, halved

¼ cup (1 oz) dried cranberries or dried apricots, chopped

scant ½ cup (2 oz) toasted slivered almonds

3½ bars (5 oz) milk chocolate (see box, page 19)

Preheat the oven to 350°F (180°C). Line two baking sheets with parchment paper (you will need to bake these in batches).

Place the butter, sugar, and honey in a medium nonstick pan over low heat. When the butter has melted, add the flour, and keep stirring for about 3 minutes, until the mixture has melted to a smooth, golden paste. Remove the pan from the heat, and fold in the fruit and nuts.

Use a couple of teaspoons to shape the mixture into small heaps on the baking sheets. Space out to allow for spreading, and then flatten each one slightly. Bake for about 8–10 minutes, until they are a mid-golden caramel colour.

Leave the cookies to harden and cool on the baking sheet for about 10–15 minutes, then transfer them to a wire rack.

Melt the chocolate in the microwave, or in a heatproof bowl set over a pan of just simmering water—don't let the bowl touch the water—and stir until smooth. Use a teaspoon to coat the flat side of each Florentine with warm melted chocolate. Just before the chocolate sets, pull a fork through in a wavy line to make a pattern on the underside.

☐ **TO STORE:** Pack the cooled Florentines between layers of parchment paper, and put into an airtight container for up to 1 week.

✱ **TO FREEZE:** Not suitable.

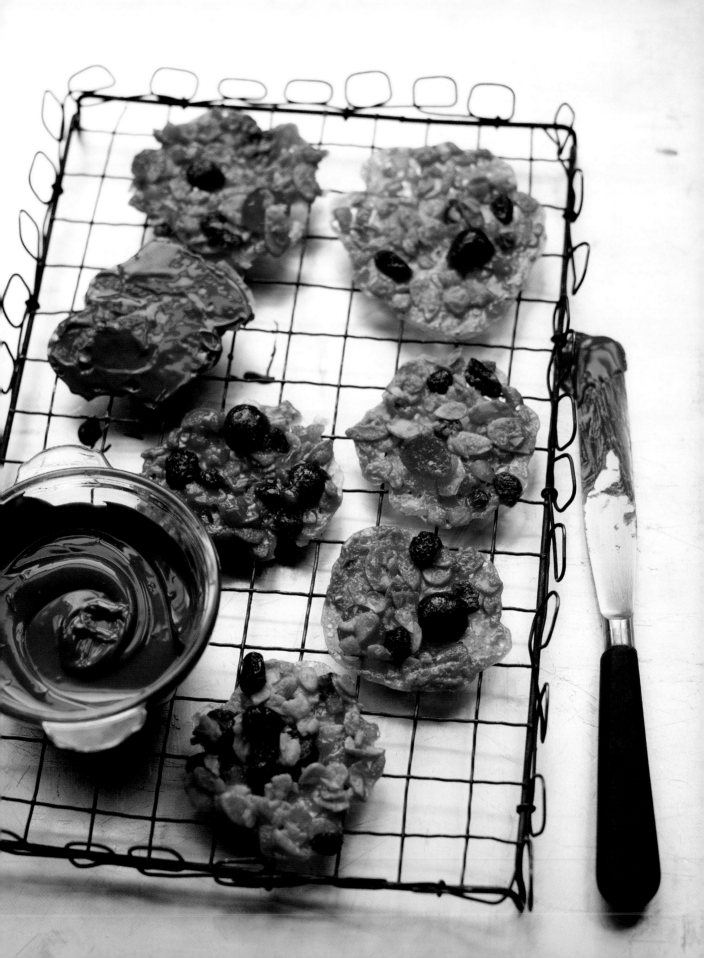

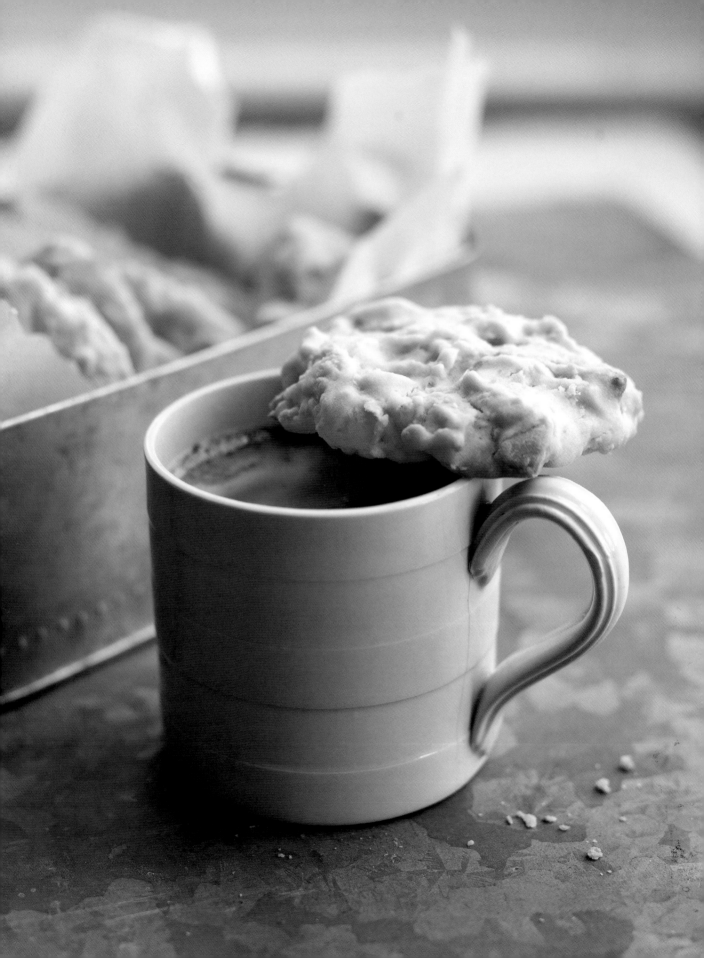

WHITE CHOC CHIP & APPLE COOKIES

This is a simple recipe, and so good to eat! The white chocolate really helps bring out the flavor of the apple, and also helps with the setting of the cookies. The grated apple needs to be squeezed out really well to get the best results. If the apple turns slightly brown, don't worry. I think it adds a nice color to the cookies.

MAKES: 12 SMALL COOKIES
PREPARATION: 15 MINUTES
BAKING: 15-20 MINUTES

---

7 tablespoons (3½ oz) margarine

1½ cups (7 oz) Gluten-Free Flour Mix A (see page 22)

¼ teaspoon baking powder (see box, page 19)

scant ½ cup (3½ oz) superfine sugar

2 large pinches ground ginger

1 large egg, at room temperature

1 medium crisp, tart apple, grated and thoroughly squeezed to extract the moisture

¾ bar (2 oz) white chocolate (see box, page 19), finely chopped

Place the margarine, flour, baking powder, sugar, and ginger in a food processor and blitz well. Add the egg, and process briefly, then transfer to a medium mixing bowl. Add the grated apple and chopped chocolate, and mix really well. Roll the dough into a 6–8-inch (15–20 cm) long cylinder, then wrap in plastic wrap and chill for 15 minutes.

Preheat the oven to 400°F (200°C). Line two baking sheets with parchment paper (you will need to bake these in batches).

Scoop off ¼-inch (5 mm) thick sections of the chilled dough with an offset spatula or spoon (you won't get neat slices because the dough will still be quite soft).

Place the cookies on the lined sheets, and bake in the oven for 15–20 minutes, or until lightly browned.

Once baked, allow the cookies to cool slightly on the sheets, then transfer to a wire rack to cool completely.

☐ **TO STORE:** Store the cooled cookies in an airtight container for up to 1 week.

✱ **TO FREEZE:** The dough and the baked cookies freeze well.
For the dough: Wrap it in plastic wrap, and freeze. Defrost for 1 hour, or until soft enough to cut and bake as above.
For the cookies: Wrap well, and store in an airtight container. Defrost for 30 minutes, then heat through at 350°F (180°C) for 2–3 minutes to soften again.

SWEET POTATO THINS

It's not often you use sweet potato in cookies, but the sweet flavor and texture make a great cookie, and it also works well in cakes.

I add a little baking powder to lighten the texture of the cookies, but the end result should be thin and crisp.

MAKES: 8–10 COOKIES
PREPARATION: 15 MINUTES
BAKING: 1 HOUR 10 MINUTES

---

1 sweet potato, approximately 4 oz

1 generous cup (5 oz) Gluten-Free Flour Mix A (see page 22)

1 teaspoon baking powder (see box, page 19)

pinch of salt

3 tablespoons superfine sugar

¼ cup (2 oz) margarine

1 large egg, at room temperature

sifted confectioners' sugar and ground allspice, for dusting

Preheat the oven to 325°F (160°C).

Bake the sweet potato for 50 minutes, until soft. Cool slightly, then peel and mash with a fork. Set the potato aside to cool completely.

Place the flour, baking powder, salt, sugar, and margarine into a medium mixing bowl, and gently rub together, or place in a food processor and pulse until you have achieved the consistency of fine bread crumbs. Add the egg and cold sweet potato, and mix well. Then roll the dough into a 6–8-inch (15–20 cm) long cylinder and chill in the fridge for at least 1 hour.

When the dough is chilled, and you are ready to bake the cookies, line a baking sheet with parchment paper (you will need to cook these in batches).

Cut the dough into ¼-inch (5 mm) slices and place on the sheet. Flatten out with your fingers until about ⅛-inch (3 mm) thick, or thinner if possible. Bake for 18–20 minutes, or until lightly browned and crisp, then leave to cool on the sheet or on a wire rack.

Serve dusted with confectioners' sugar and ground allspice

☐ **TO STORE:** Store the cooled cookies in an airtight container for up to 1 week.

✳ **TO FREEZE:** The raw dough freezes well. Wrap it in plastic wrap, and freeze. Defrost for 1 hour, or until soft enough to cut and cook as above.

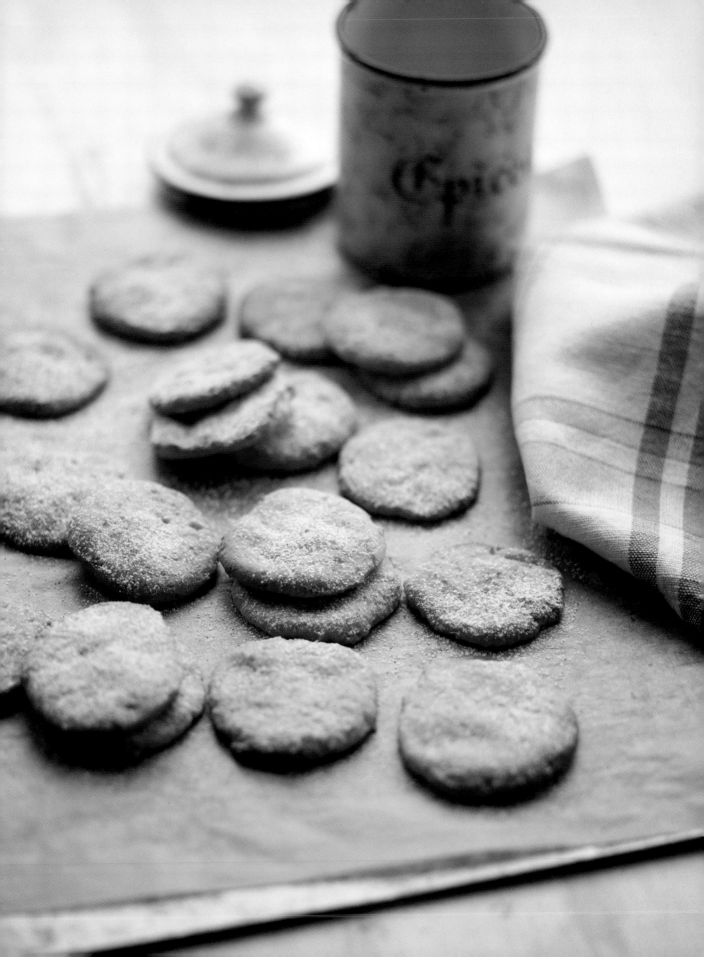

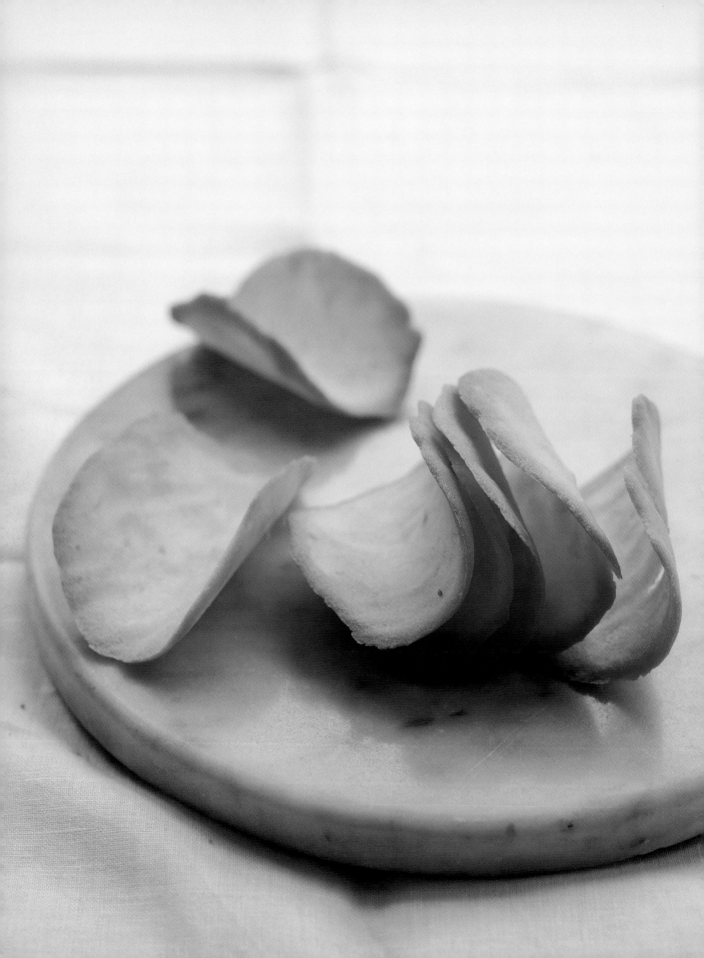

ZESTY ORANGE & ALMOND TUILES

These nice, light, crisp cookies are great to serve with ice cream and sorbets. They also look very decorative.

MAKES: ABOUT 20 TUILES
PREPARATION: 10 MINUTES
BAKING: 25 MINUTES

¾ cup (3 oz) confectioners' sugar, sifted

2 large egg whites, at room temperature

1 egg yolk, at room temperature

3 tablespoons Gluten-Free Flour Mix A (see page 22)

2 heaping tablespoons chopped or slivered almonds

2 tablespoons (1 oz) unsalted butter, melted

zest of 1 large orange

Place the sugar, egg whites, egg yolk, flour, and almonds into a bowl, and mix well. Carefully add the melted butter and orange zest, and stir well. Chill in the fridge, preferably overnight, but if you cannot wait, 3 hours minimum.

Preheat the oven to 350°F (180°C). Line two baking sheets with parchment paper (you will need to cook these in batches).

Spoon tablespoons of the mixture onto the baking sheets, and spread out with fingers wetted in cold water. Spread as thinly as possible (do not worry about any small holes), the thinner the better. Bake in the oven until the edges of the cookies start to turn a pale amber color, then remove the sheets from the oven, and allow the tuiles to cool. This is called poaching and ensures that the tuiles cook evenly. If you cook the tuiles for longer, the outsides will burn before the inside is cooked.

When the tuiles are completely cool, return the sheets to the oven, and bake for 2–3 minutes, until they are a pale golden color.

When baked, remove from the paper with an offset spatula, and lay over a rolling pin to set and cool (see picture on page 26). You may find that not all of the tuiles bake at the same time, so remove the baked tuiles one at a time, and return the sheets to the oven to allow the others to finish baking.

☐ **TO STORE:** Carefully transfer the cooled tuiles to an airtight container (or they will go soft very quickly) for up to 1 week, taking care, as they are quite fragile.

✱ **TO FREEZE:** Not suitable.

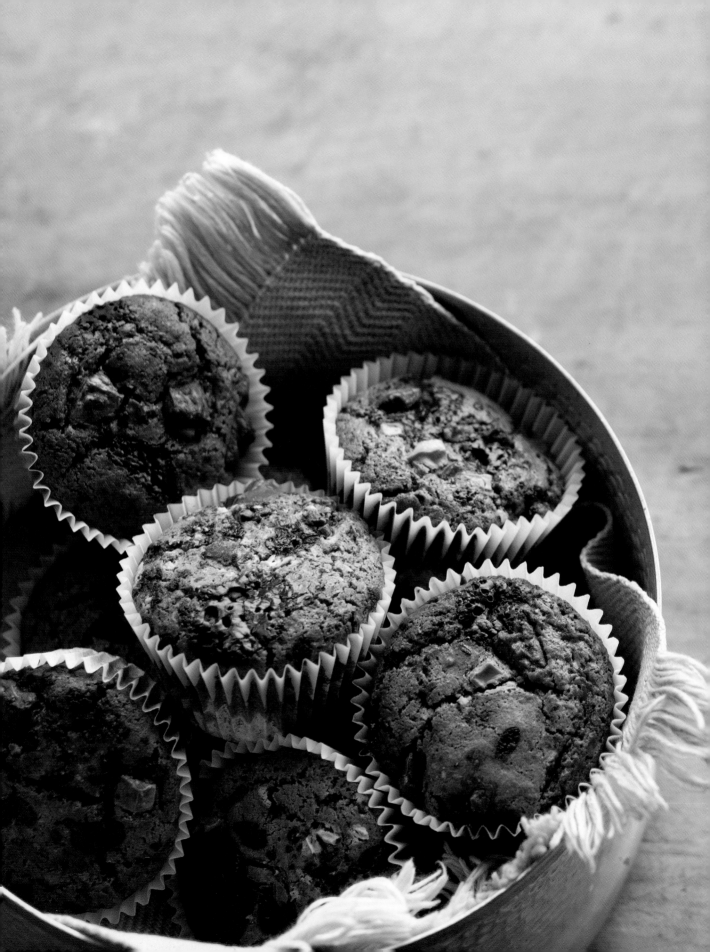

CUPCAKES & MUFFINS

HONEY MADELEINES WITH CHOCOLATE DIP

Madeleines are a traditional sweet, soft French fancy. In France they use a whisked sponge method, but here I'm using a beaten method, which works extremely well. Make sure you beat the mixture until very light and creamy before adding the egg. The mixture is flavored with a touch of honey, and the finished cakes are half dipped in chocolate and eaten warm or set—fabulous! Madeleines are perfect as an afternoon snack, or you could serve them with coffee after a meal.

MAKES: 12 CAKES
PREPARATION: 10 MINUTES
BAKING: 12–15 MINUTES

vegetable oil, for oiling

6 tablespoons superfine sugar

1 tablespoon clear honey

½ cup (4 oz) margarine, at room temperature

1 large egg, beaten, at room temperature

1 teaspoon glycerin

generous ½ cup (3 oz) Gluten-Free Flour Mix A (see page 22)

½ teaspoon baking powder (see box, page 19)

¾ cup (5 ½ oz) bittersweet chocolate (see box, page 19)

Preheat the oven to 350°F (180°C). Thoroughly oil a 12-cup tartlet pan.

In a medium bowl, whisk the sugar, honey, and margarine together really well, until very light and creamy. Gradually add the beaten egg and glycerin, stirring well after each addition. Then add the flour and baking powder, and mix well.

Spoon the mixture into the prepared pans, and bake for 12–15 minutes, until well risen and well browned. Remove the cakes from the pans, and cool on a wire rack.

Melt the chocolate in the microwave, or in a heatproof bowl set over a pan of just simmering water—don't let the bowl touch the water—and stir until smooth.

Dip half of each cake into the melted chocolate, then serve immediately, or allow to set on plastic wrap or a sheet of parchment paper.

☐ **TO STORE:** Store in an airtight container for up to 1 week.

✱ **TO FREEZE:** Once cooled, and before dipping in chocolate, freeze either in a plastic bag or an airtight container. Defrost and dip in chocolate as above before serving.

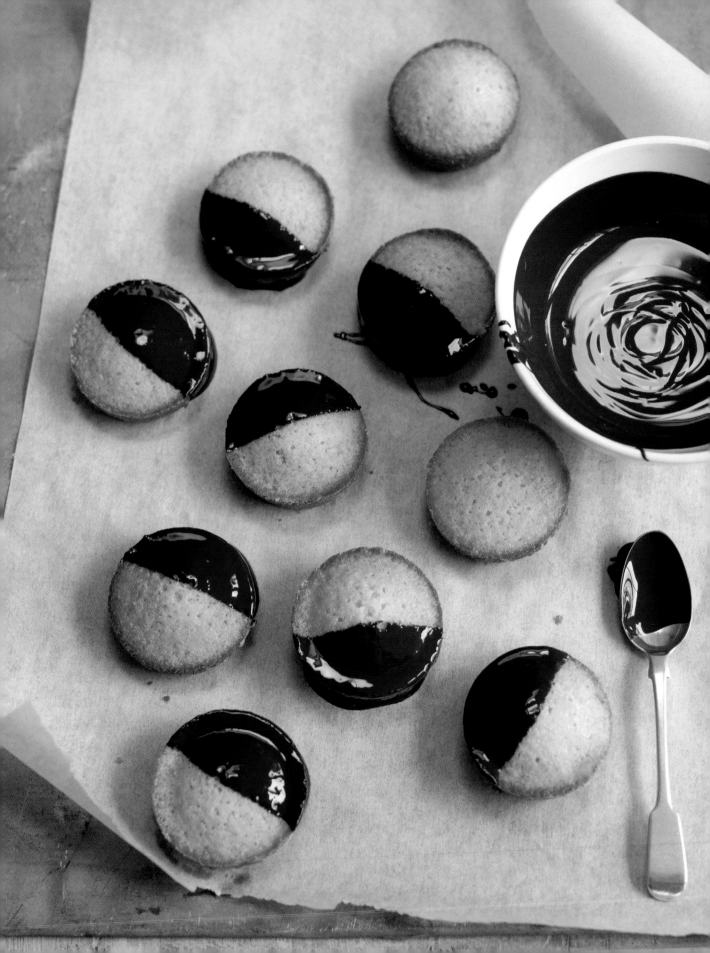

CARAMEL CHOCOLATE FUDGE BROWNIE MUFFINS

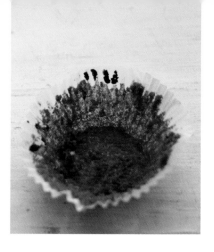

These really are wicked—gooey, sticky muffins, full of chocolate and caramel! The best thing to do is to leave them slightly underbaked, so you still have a gooey, chocolatey, caramel center. Great warm on their own or with ice cream.

MAKES: 12 MUFFINS
PREPARATION: 20 MINUTES
BAKING: 20 MINUTES

1¼ cups (6½ oz) Gluten-Free Flour Mix A (see page 22)

¼ cup (2 oz) dark brown sugar

¼ cup (2 oz) superfine sugar

3 tablespoons cocoa powder

2 teaspoons baking powder (see box, page 19)

1 large egg, at room temperature

1 teaspoon vanilla extract

1¼ cups (14 oz) dulce de leche, from a jar or can

2½ tablespoons (1 oz) each of bittersweet, milk and white chocolate (see box, page 19), chopped

Preheat the oven to 350°F (180°C). Place 12 paper muffin liners in a muffin pan.

Place the flour, sugars, cocoa, and baking powder in a bowl, and mix together well. Next place the egg, vanilla extract, and half the dulce de leche in a separate bowl, and mix together well.

Add the egg mixture to the flour and sugar, and mix well, then add the chopped chocolate and the rest of the dulce de leche, and carefully "chop" through with a spoon, leaving the mixture roughly combined. Spoon into the muffin liners, and bake in the oven for 18–20 minutes.

Remove when well risen and still slightly underbaked. Cool slightly on a wire rack, and eat warm or cold.

☐ **TO STORE:** Store in an airtight container for up to 1 week.

✱ **TO FREEZE:** Once cooled, freeze either in a plastic bag or an airtight container. Defrost for 1 hour, then warm each muffin through for 10 seconds in the microwave on full power.

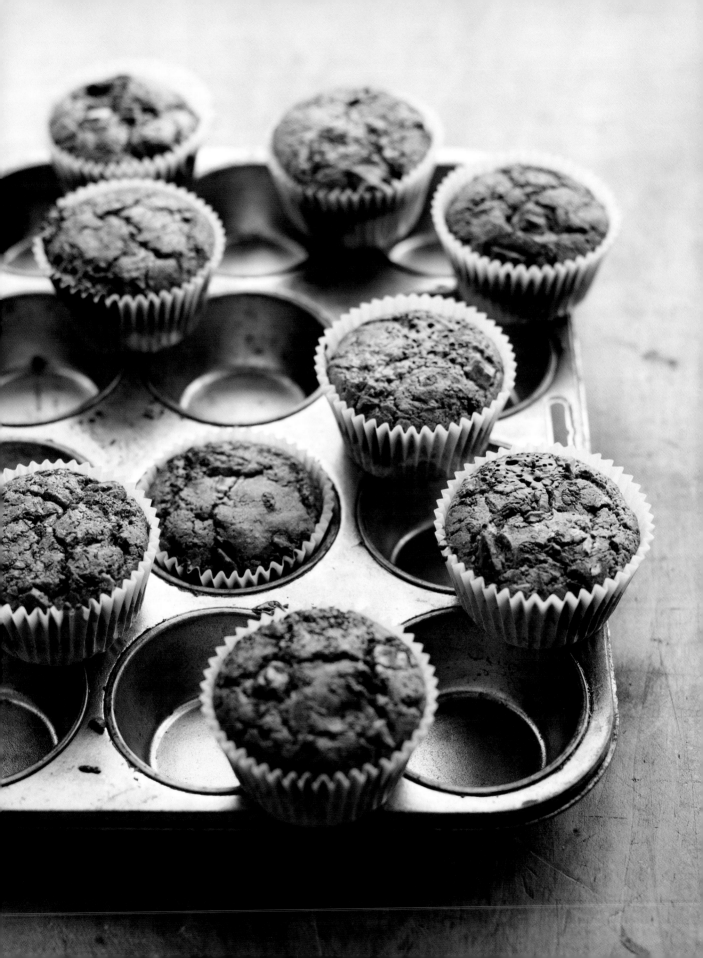

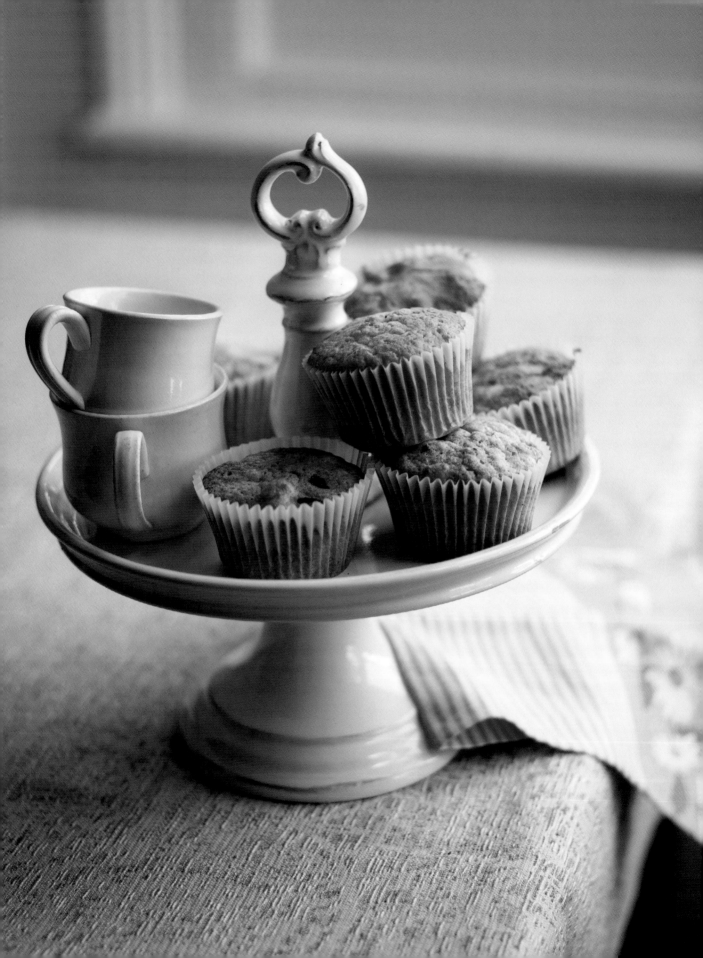

ROASTED SWEET POTATO & CHOCOLATE MUFFINS

The best way to cook sweet potatoes for recipes like this is to bake them for about 50 minutes. The flesh will shrink away from the skin, and the reduction of the original raw volume will sweeten and intensify the flavor of the sweet potato. This also reduces the amount of water in the potato, so you can get away with using only a little xanthan gum to help the finished texture.

MAKES: 12 MUFFINS
PREPARATION: 15 MINUTES
BAKING: 1 HOUR 10 MINUTES

About 7 oz sweet potatoes

2 large eggs, at room
  temperature

⅔ cup (5½ oz) superfine sugar

1½ cups (7 oz) Gluten-Free Flour
  Mix A (see page 22)

2 teaspoons baking powder
  (see box, page 19)

½ teaspoon xanthan gum

⅔ cup (5 fl oz) mild olive oil

1 teaspoon glycerin

2 tablespoons (¾ oz) each
  of bittersweet and white
  chocolate (see box, page 19)

Preheat the oven to 325°F (160°C). Place 12 paper muffin liners in a muffin pan.

Bake the sweet potato for 50 minutes, until soft. Cool slightly, then peel and mash with a fork. Set the potato aside to cool completely.

Increase the oven temperature to 350°F (180°C).

Place the eggs and sugar in a stand mixer, and beat on high speed until thick and foamy, about 5 minutes. Place the flour, baking powder, and xanthan gum in a separate bowl, and mix well. Whisk the oil and glycerin together in a small bowl.

Add the sweet potato flesh to the flour mixture, and chop through with a spoon or fork, breaking it up so the mixture is roughly combined. Roughly chop the bittersweet and white chocolate, and stir into the mixture.

Add the oil mix to the eggs, along with the flour and sweet potato; mix well, but lightly.

Spoon the mixture into the muffin liners and bake for 20 minutes, or until well risen and lightly browned.

Remove the muffin pan from the oven, and let cool on a wire rack.

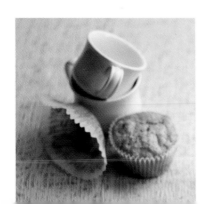

☐ **TO STORE:** Store in an airtight container for up to 1 week.

✳ **TO FREEZE:** Once cooled, freeze in a plastic bag or an airtight container.

BLUEBERRY BUTTERMILK MUFFINS

A tasty twist on a much used format, here the frozen blueberries defrost perfectly when baking, leaving little pockets of brilliantly purple juice. Don't restrict yourself to blueberries though—any frozen berries will work.

Soaking the oats in buttermilk first really helps keep the muffins moist. Buttermilk is the by-product when butter is produced; it has a slight acidic edge to it, and this, coupled with the baking soda and baking powder, causes a slight chemical reaction, producing bubbles of air to increase the lift in the end result—all clever stuff!

MAKES: 12 MUFFINS
PREPARATION: 15 MINUTES
BAKING: 15–20 MINUTES

2⅓ cups (7 oz) rolled oats
   (see box, page 19)

1¼ cups (10 fl oz) buttermilk

generous ½ cup (4½ oz)
   superfine sugar

⅔ cup (5 fl oz) vegetable oil

1 large egg, at room
   temperature

1 tablespoon glycerin

1½ cups (7 oz) Gluten-Free Flour
   Mix A (see page 22)

1½ teaspoons baking powder
   (see box, page 19)

½ teaspoon xanthan gum

½ teaspoon baking soda

scant ½ cup (3 oz) frozen
   blueberries

Preheat the oven to 400°F (200°C). Place 12 paper muffin liners in a muffin pan.

Place the oats, buttermilk, and sugar in a medium mixing bowl, and set aside for 20 minutes.

Whisk the oil, egg, and glycerin together in a bowl, and add to the oat mixture. Then stir in the flour, baking powder, xanthan gum, and baking soda. Finally add the blueberries, and mix well.

Spoon into the muffin liners and bake for 15 minutes, or until well browned and risen.

Cool on a wire rack, and serve.

☐ **TO STORE:** Store in an airtight container for up to 1 week.

✱ **TO FREEZE:** Once cooled, freeze either in a plastic bag or an airtight container.

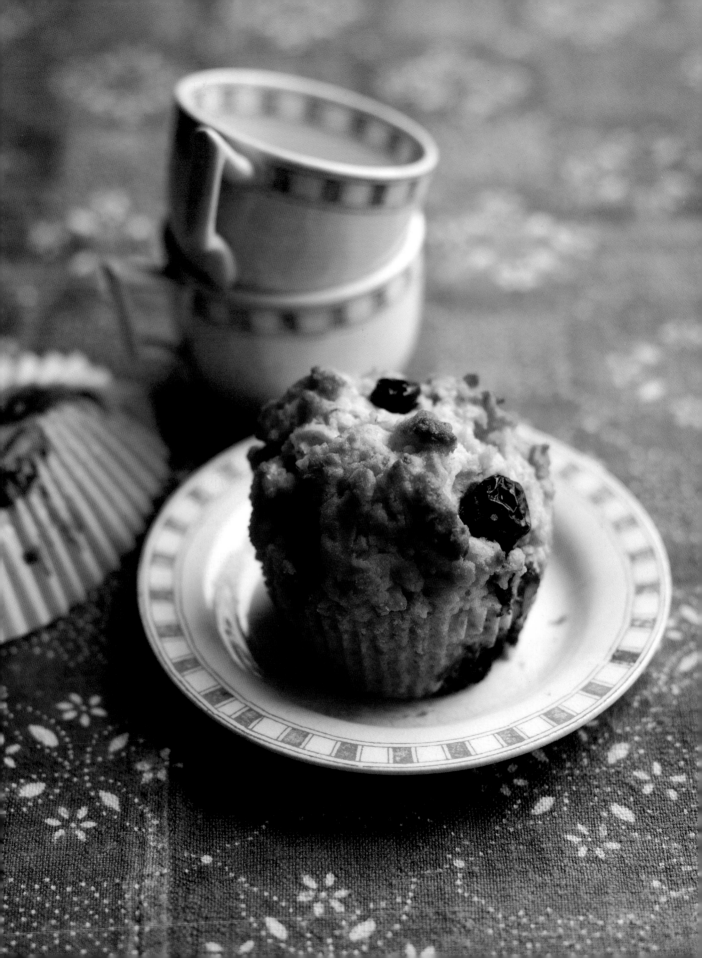

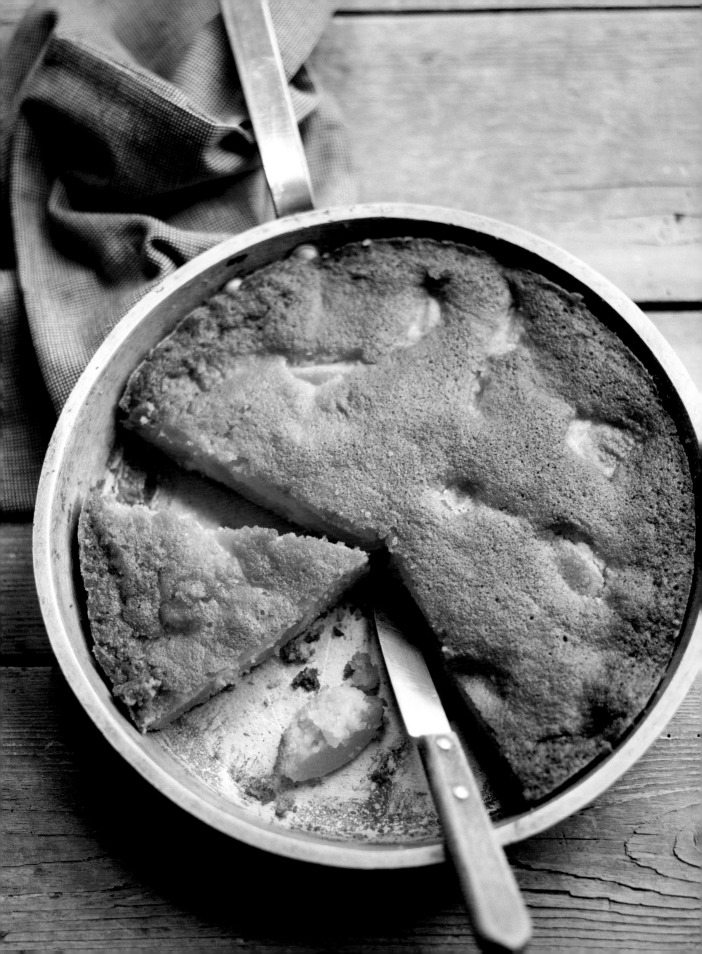

EASY APRICOT & BRANDY PAN MUFFIN

Muffins are generally made in small individual pans. But this is a fruity muffin recipe with a difference—all you need is an ovenproof non-stick skillet to cook it in!

A couple of good tips here: make sure the margarine and eggs are at room temperature (warming the mixing bowl makes it easier to cream them together too). And warm the milk with the glycerin. This will ensure the mixture won't curdle or split, making a lighter, more even-textured sponge. It will also ensure the maximum lift from the sponge when baking. Glycerin helps to retain moisture in the cake's structure; something that's essential when cooking without gluten.

MAKES: ONE 10-INCH (25 CM) ROUND, 2-INCH (5 CM) DEEP MUFFIN
PREPARATION: 15 MINUTES
BAKING: 20-30 MINUTES

1¼ cups (6¼ oz) Gluten-Free Flour Mix A (see page 22)

1 teaspoon baking soda

1 teaspoon baking powder (see box, page 19)

6 tablespoons (3 oz) margarine, at room temperature

⅔ cup (5 oz) superfine sugar

2 large eggs, at room temperature

generous ½ cup (4 fl oz) 2% milk, warmed with 1 teaspoon glycerin

2–3 tablespoons brandy

2 tablespoons vegetable oil

2 × 15-oz cans apricot halves in syrup, drained

Preheat the oven to 350°F (180°C).

Place the flour, baking soda, and baking powder in a medium bowl, and mix well.

Warm a large mixing bowl under hot running water. Place the margarine and sugar in the bowl, and beat them together until light and creamy.

Add the flour mixture and eggs to the creamed mixture, and stir well. Then add the warm milk, glycerin and brandy, and mix to a batter consistency.

Heat a 10-inch (25cm) x 2-inch (5cm) deep nonstick ovenproof skillet over medium heat, and add the oil. Arrange the apricots evenly in the pan, round side down, cut side up. Spoon the batter over the fruit evenly, then, with an offset spatula or the back of a tablespoon, spread it over the fruit to even it out.

Bake in the oven for 20–25 minutes, or until risen and lightly colored.

Remove and cool in the pan for 5 minutes, then invert the muffin onto a wire rack to cool completely. To serve, transfer it to a plate, and cut into wedges.

☐ **TO STORE:** Store whole, or cut into wedges, in an airtight container for up to 1 week.

✱ **TO FREEZE:** Freeze on the serving plate, wrapped in foil.

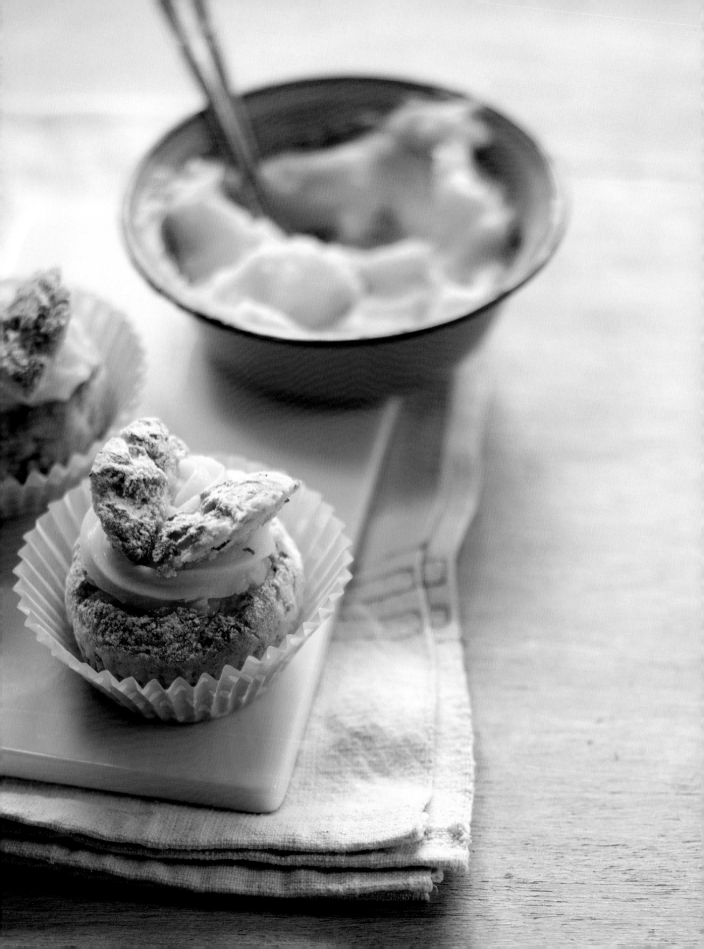

SWEET ZUCCHINI & SAFFRON BUTTERFLY CAKES

When I was a child, my mom would make butterfly cakes, and I still love them! The addition of grated zucchini and saffron gives a lovely soft edge to these cakes. Good old-fashioned buttercream (now more commonly known as frosting) is a lovely way to finish them.

MAKES: 12 CAKES
PREPARATION: 20 MINUTES
BAKING: 15–20 MINUTES

- 1 good pinch saffron threads or powder

- 2 tablespoons boiling water

- 2 large eggs, at room temperature

- generous ¾ cup (6½ oz) superfine sugar

- 1½ cups (7 oz) Gluten-Free Flour Mix A (see page 22)

- 2 teaspoons baking powder (see box, page 19)

- ½ teaspoon xanthan gum

- 1 teaspoon glycerin

- 2 medium zucchini, grated and thoroughly squeezed to extract the moisture

- 1 cup (8 oz) unsalted butter, softened

- ⅔ cup (2½ oz) confectioners' sugar, sifted

- sifted confectioners' sugar, to dust

Preheat the oven to 350°F (180°C). Place 12 paper muffin liners in a muffin pan.

Place the saffron threads or powder in a mug, add the boiling water, and leave to infuse and cool.

Next, place the eggs and sugar into a stand mixer, and beat on high speed for 5 minutes, or until thick and creamy.

Place the flour, baking powder, and xanthan gum together in another bowl, and mix well.

Once the egg and sugar are very thick, add the saffron water, glycerin, flour mix, and zucchini. Fold together well, then spoon into the muffin liners.

Bake for 15–20 minutes, until slightly brown and well risen. Remove, and allow to cool completely on a wire rack.

To make the buttercream, beat the butter and confectioners' sugar together in a medium bowl.

Once the cakes are cold, cut out a small, fairly deep circle of cake from the top of each muffin with a sharp knife, then cut each circle in half. Spoon a little frosting into the hole in the cake, then invert the two half circles of cake, and stick onto the frosting to simulate butterfly wings.

Dust with confectioners' sugar, and serve.

For a splash more color
Try adding a little infused saffron (1 small pinch of saffron threads or powder infused in 2 teaspoons boiling water) to the buttercream for extra color.

☐ **TO STORE:** Store, unfrosted, in an airtight container for up to 1 week.

✱ **TO FREEZE:** Once cooled, freeze the unfrosted cakes in a plastic bag or airtight container.

COFFEE CUPCAKES WITH MOCHA FONDANT FROSTING

This frosting is delicious, and makes these really special. I use fondant icing sugar, which is available from some specialist markets and online. You can also make your own (see page 40).

MAKES: 12 CUPCAKES
PREPARATION: 10 MINUTES
BAKING: 20 MINUTES

For the cupcakes

1¼ cups (6¼ oz) Gluten-Free Flour Mix A or B (see page 22)

1½ teaspoons baking powder (see box, page 19)

½ teaspoon xanthan gum

generous ¾ cup (6¼ oz) superfine sugar

2 large eggs, at room temperature

1 teaspoon vanilla extract

1 teaspoon glycerin

½ cup (4 fl oz) 2% milk

½ cup (4 fl oz) sunflower oil

2 tablespoons instant coffee dissolved in 1 tablespoon boiling water

For the mocha fondant frosting

1 tablespoon instant coffee and 2 teaspoons cocoa powder dissolved in 2 tablespoons boiling water

1¼ cups (5½ oz) fondant icing sugar

Preheat the oven to 350°F (180°C). Place 12 paper muffin liners in a muffin pan.

Mix the flour, baking powder, and xanthan gum together.

Place the superfine sugar, eggs, vanilla, and glycerin in another mixing bowl and, using a hand-held electric mixer, beat on high speed for a couple of minutes until thick and double in volume. When the eggs are nice and thick, fold in the flour mix.

Next, mix the milk and the oil with the coffee liquid in a bowl. Start beating on low speed, and slowly pour the liquid into the cake batter; beat well, but don't go mad. It will still seem quite wet. Divide the batter between the 12 liners, filling them about half full.

Bake for about 20 minutes, or until well risen and a toothpick inserted into the center comes out clean. Remove, and allow to cool completely on a wire rack.

To make the frosting, mix the mocha liquid gradually into the fondant icing sugar; add more or less liquid to make a thick paste. Spread the frosting onto the center of each cold cupcake, and coax it to the sides. The fondant frosting gives a brilliant shine to the topping for the cupcakes.

Topping variation
You could skip the cocoa in the icing; top with a glistening coffee glaze, and sprinkle with some crushed walnuts for a retro coffee and walnut taste.

☐ **TO STORE:** Store, unfrosted, in an airtight container for up to 1 week.

✱ **TO FREEZE:** Once cooled, freeze the unfrosted cakes in a plastic bag or airtight container.

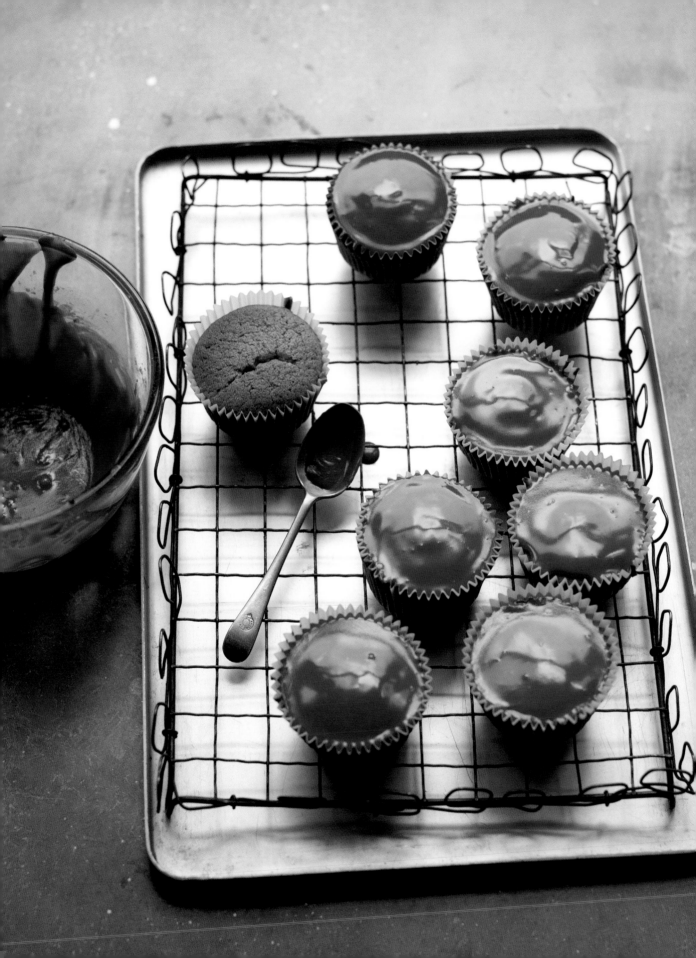

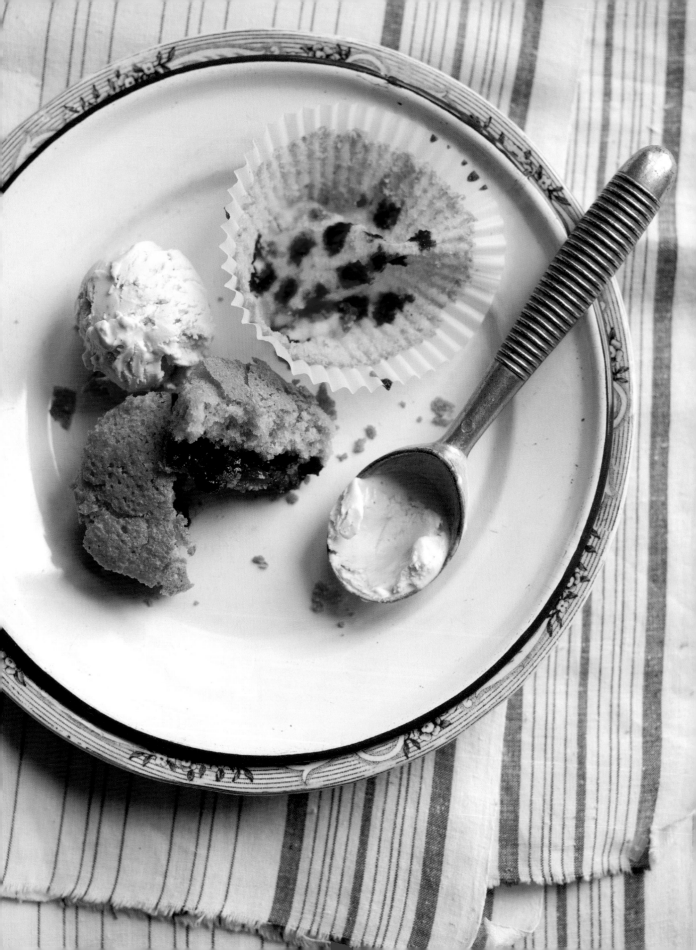

TANGY BEET & BLACK CURRANT MUFFINS

The use of sweet pickled beets, along with the black currants, makes a nice difference, giving an almost sweet and sour edge to these muffins. They are delicious served warm with a scoop of vanilla ice cream, and I have also been known to eat them warm with a slice of Gorgonzola cheese or a sliver of mature Cheddar cheese! You may have to substitute other berries if black currants are not available.

MAKES: 12 MUFFINS
PREPARATION: 15 MINUTES
BAKING: 15–18 MINUTES

---

2 large eggs, at room
  temperature

1 cup (8 oz) superfine sugar

1¼ cups (6¼ oz) Gluten-Free
  Flour Mix A (see page 22)

pinch of salt

1½ teaspoons baking powder
  (see box, page 19)

generous ½ cup (4 fl oz)
  vegetable oil

generous ½ cup (4 fl oz)
  2% milk

1 teaspoon glycerin

generous ½ cup (3½ oz) sweet
  pickled beets, drained and
  finely diced

½ cup (3½ oz) frozen black
  currants, blackberries, or
  other berries

Preheat the oven to 350°F (180°C). Place 12 paper muffin liners in a muffin pan.

Whisk the eggs and sugar in a medium bowl for about 2 minutes by hand.

Mix all the dry ingredients really well together. Combine the oil, milk, and glycerin in a bowl. Add the dry ingredients to the beaten eggs and sugar, followed by the oil mixture, then mix well. Next stir in the beets and black currants.

Scoop the mixture into the muffin liners, and bake for 15–18 minutes, or until well risen and baked through. Remove and allow to cool on a wire rack.

☐ **TO STORE:** Store in an airtight container for up to 1 week.

✳ **TO FREEZE:** Once cooled, freeze in a plastic bag or airtight container.

BLUE CHEESE BUTTERMILK MUFFINS

A savory version of the ever-popular muffin that is light, tasty, and really easy to make, and they also freeze really well. You can use any blue cheese for this recipe, such as Stilton, or you could try dolcelatte for a lighter texture.

MAKES: 10 MUFFINS
PREPARATION: 15 MINUTES
BAKING: 20–25 MINUTES

---

2 cups (8 oz) Gluten-Free Flour Mix B (see page 22)

2 teaspoons baking powder (see box, page 19)

pinch of celery salt

½ cup (2 oz) blue cheese, crumbled or finely chopped

small handful of fresh basil leaves, snipped

¾ cup (6 fl oz) 2% milk

scant ½ cup (3½ fl oz) buttermilk

4 tablespoons (2 oz) unsalted butter, melted

1 extra large egg, at room temperature

Preheat the oven to 400°F (200°C). Prepare a muffin pan: cut 10 squares of wax paper, one for each cup, with the edges overlapping, or line with 10 paper muffin liners.

Sift the flour into a large bowl with the baking powder and celery salt. Stir in the cheese and the basil.

In a large bowl, beat the milks, melted butter, and egg together with a hand-held electric mixer.

Make a well in the center of the dry ingredients, and gradually add the liquid ingredients. The mixture should be soft, but not too thick. Immediately spoon the mixture into the muffin liners, filling them about half full.

Bake for 20–25 minutes, or until well risen and golden. Remove and eat when still warm, or allow to cool on a wire rack.

Variation
For an extra burst of flavor, add 5–6 sun-dried tomatoes packed in oil. Drain well, finely chop, and add to the mixture at the same time as the cheese.

☐ **TO STORE:** Store in an airtight container for up to 1 week. Warm the cold muffins for a few seconds in a microwave before serving.

✳ **TO FREEZE:** Once cooled, double wrap in plastic wrap and freeze in an airtight container. Defrost for 1 hour, and then warm each muffin through for 10 seconds in the microwave on full power.

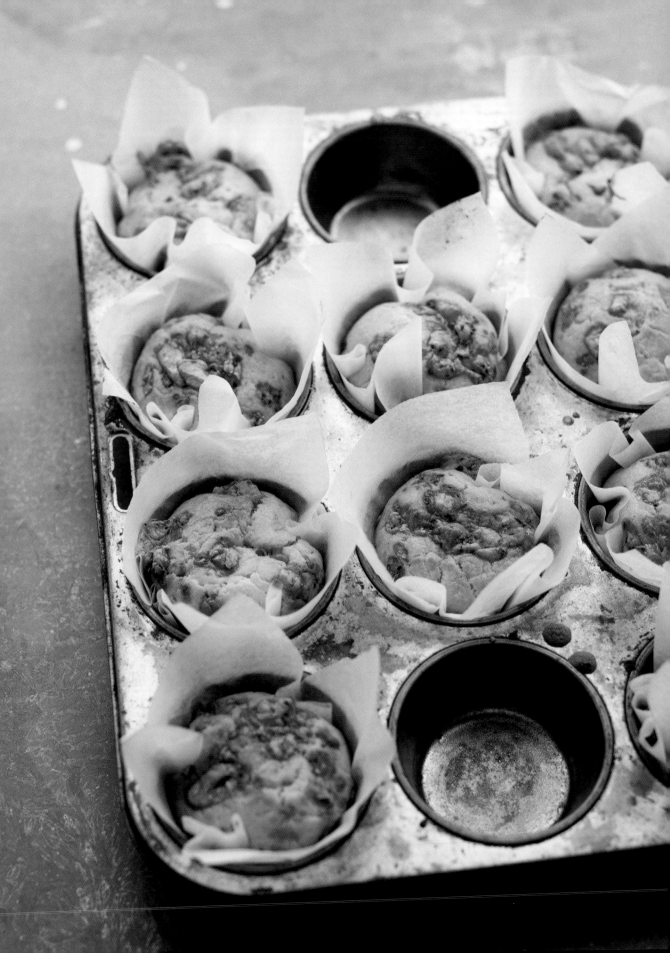

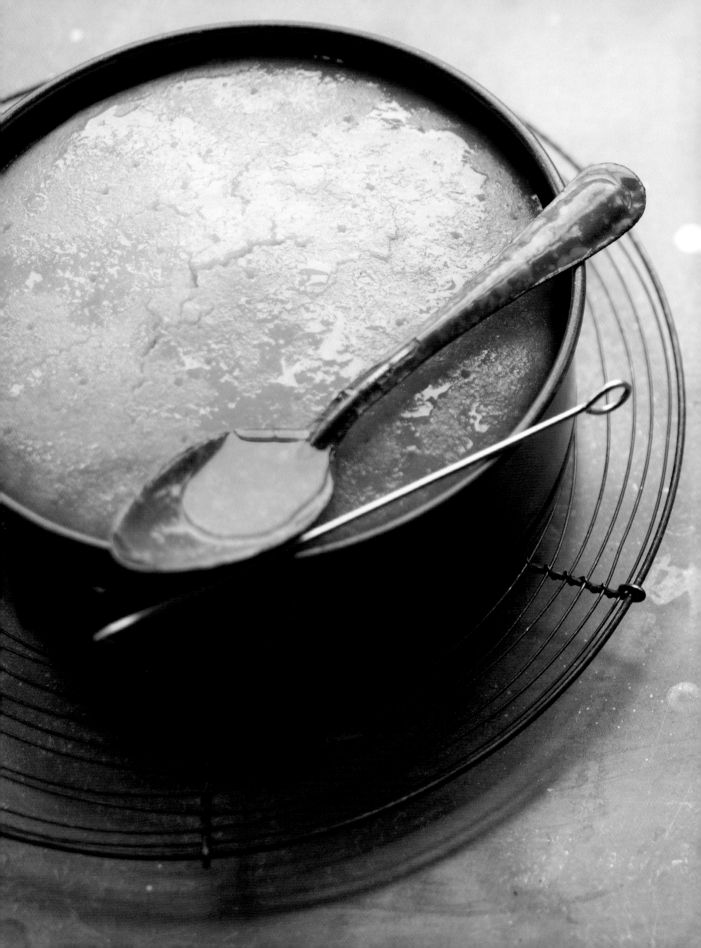

LARGE CAKES

POLENTA CAKE WITH RASPBERRY DRIZZLE FROSTING

Polenta cakes are very trendy at the moment—there's hardly a week goes by when you don't see a recipe in the weekend newspapers. Here is a light-textured version—bear in mind the finer the cornmeal, the smoother the texture of the cake. I quite like a grittier texture.

MAKES: ONE 8-INCH (20 CM)
   SQUARE CAKE
PREPARATION: 10 MINUTES
BAKING: 45–50 MINUTES

For the sponge cake

vegetable oil, for oiling

¾ cup (6¼ oz) unsalted butter, softened

1 cup (8 oz) superfine sugar

3 large eggs, at room temperature

1 generous cup (5½ oz) fine cornmeal (see box, page 19)

¾ cup (3½ oz) Gluten-Free Flour Mix A (see page 22)

2 teaspoons xanthan gum

1 tablespoon glycerin

½ teaspoon baking powder (see box, page 19)

For the frosting

finely grated zest and juice of 2 large limes

2¼ cups (9 oz) fondant icing sugar (see page 40)

scant 2 cups (9 oz) fresh or frozen raspberries

Preheat the oven to 350°F (180°C). Lightly oil a 2½-inch (6 cm) deep, 8-inch (20 cm) square cake pan with a removable bottom.

Lightly cream the butter and sugar together in a large mixing bowl. Beat in the eggs, cornmeal, flour, xanthan gum, glycerin, and baking powder. Stir well, and pour into the prepared cake pan.

Place the pan on a baking sheet, and bake for 40–45 minutes, or until well risen and lightly browned.

Remove from the oven and allow to cool in the pan. Then remove from the pan and place on a serving plate.

For the frosting, mix the lime juice, zest, and fondant icing sugar together until you have the consistency of very thick cream.

If using fresh raspberries, spoon the frosting over the cake, then place the raspberries on top. Leave the cake to set at room temperature.

If using frozen raspberries, coat the cake well with the frosting, place the frozen raspberries on top, and leave for 40 minutes to defrost. The juice will run into the icing and look wonderful.

☐ **TO STORE:** The unfrosted cake will keep for 1 week, stored in an airtight container.

✱ **TO FREEZE:** Freeze the cake before frosting it. Wrap it well, and place in an airtight container. Top with the frosting and raspberries once defrosted.

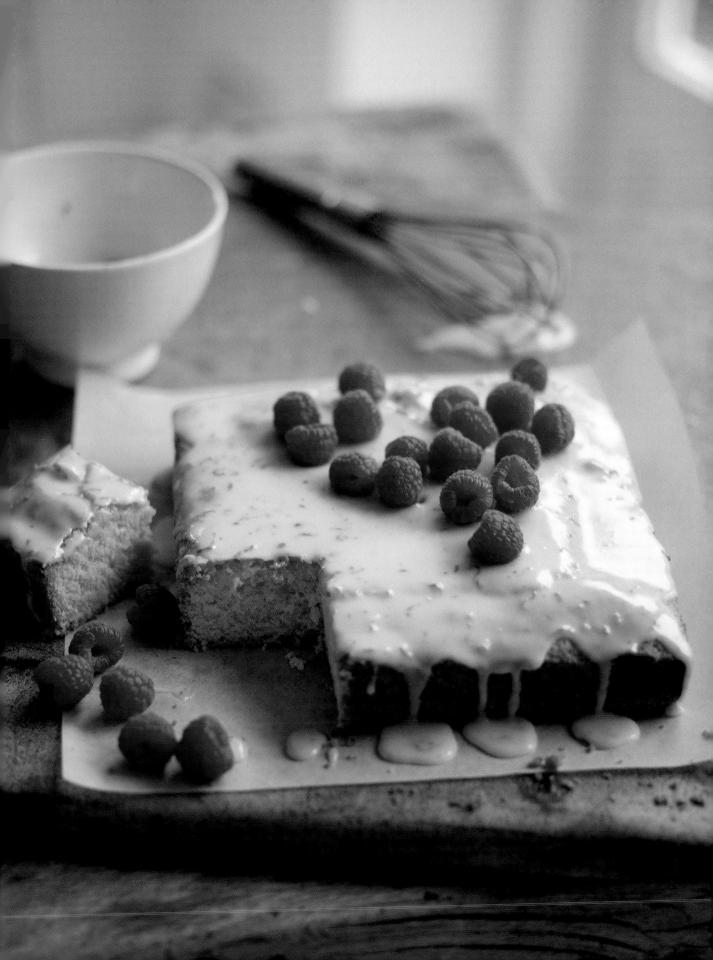

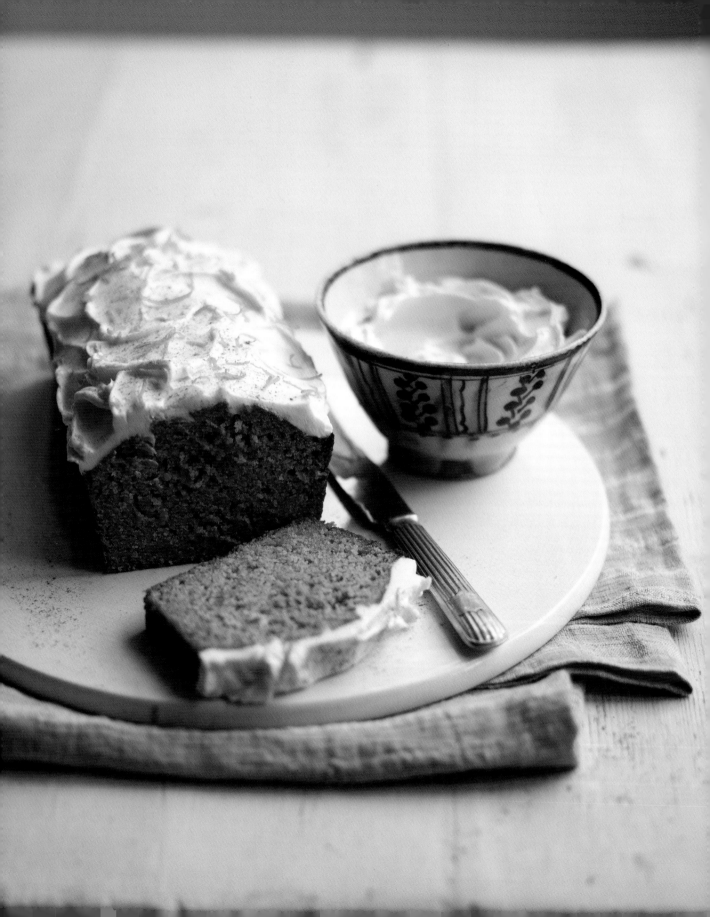

FROSTED CARROT CAKE

A twist on an old favorite here; this has a really nice texture that I reckon is better than when made with ordinary flour.

MAKES: ONE 9 × 5-INCH
   (23 × 13 CM, 2 LB) LOAF
PREPARATION: 15 MINUTES
BAKING: 40–45 MINUTES

For the carrot cake

vegetable oil, for oiling

⅔ cup (5½ oz) light brown
   sugar

generous ½ cup (4 fl oz)
   sunflower oil

3 large eggs, at room
   temperature

2 cups (8 oz) Gluten-Free Flour
   Mix B (see page 22)

1 teaspoon xanthan gum

½ teaspoon baking soda

½ teaspoon baking powder
   (see box, page 19)

½ teaspoon pumpkin pie spice

2 tablespoons 2% milk

2½ cups (9 oz) carrots, grated

For the cinnamon frosting

scant cup (7 oz) light cream
   cheese, at room temperature

¾ cup (3 oz) confectioners'
   sugar, sifted

½ teaspoon ground cinnamon

grated zest of 1 small lime or
   orange, plus extra to decorate

Preheat the oven to 350°F (180°C). Oil a 9 × 5-inch (23 × 13 cm, 2lb) loaf pan and line base with parchment paper.

Tip the sugar into a large mixing bowl. Using a hand-held electric mixer, whisk in the oil and the eggs, one at a time.

Sift together the flour, xanthan gum, baking soda, baking powder, and pumpkin pie spice, and add this to the bowl, stirring well. Add the milk, and stir well to loosen the mixture. Stir in the grated carrots, and mix all the ingredients evenly.

Spoon the mixture into the prepared pan, and bake for 40–45 minutes, until firm and springy in the center and a toothpick inserted into the center comes out clean. Cool in the pan for 10 minutes. Turn the cake out of the pan, peel off the paper, and allow to cool completely on a wire rack.

To make the frosting, beat all the ingredients together in a small bowl until smooth. Set the cake on a serving plate, spread with the frosting, sprinkle with the extra lime or orange zest, and cut into slices to serve.

Variation: carrot cupcakes

Divide the mixture between 10–12 muffin pans, then bake for 20–25 minutes, or until risen, golden, and a toothpick comes out clean when inserted into the center. Allow to cool completely on a wire rack. When cool, spread the tops with the cinnamon frosting, and decorate with lime or orange zest.

☐ **TO STORE:** The frosted cake keeps well for 2–3 days in an airtight container in the fridge.

✳ **TO FREEZE:** The unfrosted cake freezes well. Wrap the cake in parchment paper, and place it in an airtight container. Store for up to 3 months, and ice the cake after defrosting.

PEAR & BLUEBERRY POLENTA CAKE

The fruit flavors work really well in this sponge cake, which has an indulgent cream cheese frosting. You can use this as a basic recipe and change the fruit depending on what's in season. I've also given an alternative fondant frosting topping below.

MAKES: 12 SQUARES
PREPARATION: 25 MINUTES
BAKING: 30 MINUTES

For the sponge cake

vegetable oil, for oiling

3 pears

finely grated zest of 1 large lemon, plus 1 tablespoon lemon juice

¾ cup (6¼ oz) unsalted butter

1 cup (8 oz) superfine sugar

3 large eggs, beaten, at room temperature

1 teaspoon vanilla extract

1 tablespoon baking powder (see box, page 19)

scant 2 cups (9 oz) fine cornmeal (see box, page 19)

1 cup (3½ oz) blueberries

For the frosting

2 tablespoons (1 oz) butter, softened

1¼ cups (10 oz) light cream cheese

½ cup (2 oz) confectioners' sugar, sifted

Preheat the oven to 350°F (180°C). Oil a 9-inch (23 cm) square baking pan.

Pare and slice the pears, cut into rough chunks, and coat in the lemon juice to prevent them from browning.

Place the unsalted butter and superfine sugar in a mixing bowl, and cream them together, using a hand-held electric mixer. Add the eggs, half the lemon zest, the vanilla extract, baking powder, and cornmeal and mix well. Carefully fold in the pears. Spoon the mixture into the prepared pan, and press a layer of blueberries on the top.

Bake for about 30 minutes, until well risen and golden. Test with a toothpick, which should come out clean when inserted into the center. Remove from the oven and leave to cool in the pan.

For the frosting, put the butter and cream cheese into a medium bowl, mix until soft and smooth, then beat in the confectioners' sugar. Remove the cake from the pan. Spread the frosting evenly over the cake, and sprinkle with the reserved lemon zest. Cut into squares to serve. The cake is best eaten on the same day that you ice and decorate it.

Alternative fondant frosting topping

Prepare the cake as above, transfer it to the oiled pan, and bake it without the blueberries. Leave to cool in the pan.

In a medium bowl, mix 4 tablespoons of lemon juice with 2¼ cups (9 oz) fondant icing sugar (see page 40), until it is the consistency of very thick cream. Remove the cake from the pan, and spoon half the icing over the cooled cake. Top with ½ cup (2 oz) blueberries or seasonal berries of your choice. Drizzle with the rest of the frosting and leave to set.

☐ **TO STORE:** The uniced cake will keep for 2 days in an airtight container.

✱ **TO FREEZE:** Not suitable.

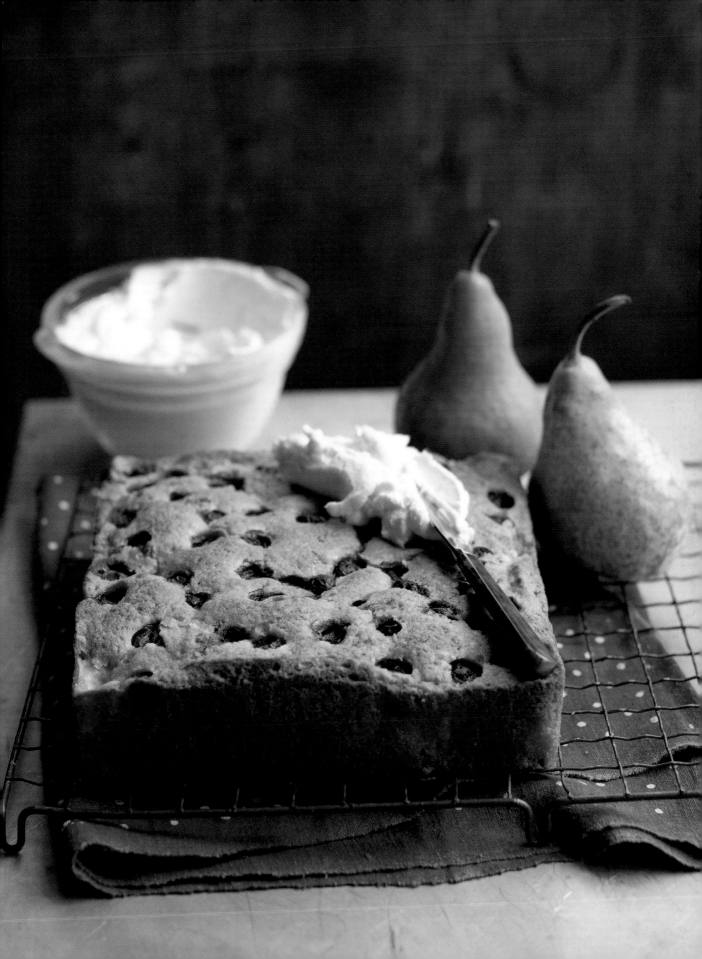

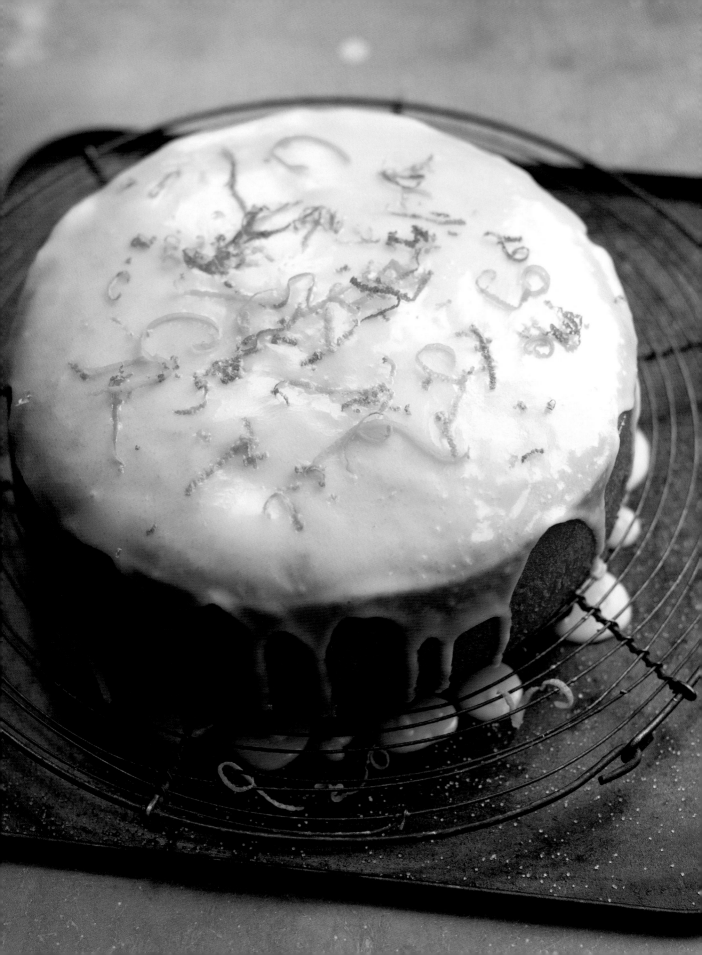

GLAZED LEMON & LIME DRIZZLE CAKE

A great tea-time favorite! I use a lemon and lime syrup to moisten the cake, and a thin lime fondant glaze to finish the cake off, which gives it a really zingy flavor.

MAKES: ONE 8-INCH (20 CM) ROUND CAKE
PREPARATION: 20 MINUTES
BAKING: 30 MINUTES, PLUS COOLING

For the cake

vegetable oil, for oiling

1 cup (8 oz) superfine sugar

4 large eggs, at room temperature

3 cups (12½ oz) Gluten-Free Flour Mix B (see page 22)

1½ teaspoons xanthan gum

2 teaspoons baking powder (see box, page 19)

1⅔ cups (13 fl oz) 2% milk

generous ¾ cup (6½ fl oz) sunflower oil

zest and juice of 2 large lemons

For the syrup

2 large limes

6 tablespoons granulated sugar

For the crunchy glaze

juice of 1 large lime

scant cup (3½ oz) fondant icing sugar (see page 40)

granulated sugar, for sprinkling

lemon and lime zest, to decorate

Preheat the oven to 350°F (180°F). Oil an 8-inch round cake pan with a removable bottom, and line base with parchment paper.

Whisk the sugar and the eggs together in a food processor until thick and creamy. Sift together the flour, xanthan gum, and baking powder to combine evenly, and add this to the sugar and eggs. Whisk in the milk, oil, and lemon zest (reserve the juice for the syrup).

Spoon the mixture into the prepared pan, and bake for about 30 minutes, until firm and springy in the center. Test with a toothpick; if it comes out clean, it's done. The cake will be nicely browned and domed. Once baked, remove from the oven, and allow it to cool slightly in the pan.

To make the syrup, squeeze the limes, and pour the juice into a measuring cup with the reserved lemon juice—you'll need approximately ½ cup (4 fl oz) in total. Next, place the measured lemon and lime juice into a small pan with the granulated sugar, and boil them together for 1 minute.

Prick the warm cake all over with a skewer while it is still in the pan, then pour on the hot syrup. Once the cake is cool, carefully remove it from the pan and place it on a wire rack to cool completely.

To make the glaze, place the lime juice in a small bowl, and add the fondant icing sugar to make a runny icing. Sprinkle the top of the cake with a little granulated sugar. Pour the icing all over the cake, and leave to run over the edges. Decorate with lemon and lime zest.

☐ **TO STORE:** The glazed cake keeps well for 2 days in an airtight container in the fridge.

✱ **TO FREEZE:** The unglazed cake freezes well. Wrap the cake in parchment paper, and place in an airtight container. Store for up to 3 months, and glaze after defrosting.

APPLE PUDDING CAKE WITH CIDER CRUNCH TOPPING

This is a cross between a cake and a bread—very moist, and absolutely delicious! The fruit gives it a dense texture, a bit like old-fashioned bread pudding, only golden in color. This is a bit of an English West Country treat, with the cider topping, especially if you serve it with generous dollops of clotted cream (which is available online and in specialty food stores)!

MAKES: ONE 8-INCH (20 CM) ROUND CAKE

PREPARATION: 20 MINUTES, PLUS 2 HOURS SOAKING TIME

BAKING: 1 HOUR

For the cake

1¼ cups (6¼ oz) mixed dried fruit

½ cup (3 oz) golden raisins

scant ½ cup (3½ fl oz) hard cider

vegetable oil, for oiling

3 cups (8 oz) Gluten-Free Flour Mix A (see page 22)

1 teaspoon xanthan gum

1 tablespoon baking powder (see box, page 19)

2 teaspoons pumpkin pie spice

¾ cup (6 oz) margarine

¾ cup (6 oz) soft light brown sugar

3 large eggs, beaten, at room temperature

3 crisp eating apples (e.g., McIntosh or Granny Smith)

For the cider crunch topping

2 tablespoons light brown sugar crystals

2 teaspoons hard cider

Place the dried fruit in a bowl, and pour the cider over. Set aside for a couple of hours to macerate.

Preheat the oven to 350°F (180°C). Oil an 8-inch (20 cm) round cake pan with a removable bottom and line base with parchment paper.

Sift the flour with the xanthan gum, baking powder, and spice. Using a hand-held electric mixer, cream the margarine and sugar together until fluffy and light. Gradually beat in the eggs, along with 2 tablespoons of the flour mixture.

Next, grate one of the apples, including the skin, into the mixture, then chop a second apple into small chunks, and fold into the cake batter along with the rest of the flour mixture. Add the soaked dried fruit and liquid, and combine the mixture well. Slice the remaining apple and reserve.

Spoon the cake mixture into the prepared pan. Press the reserved apple slices into the top of the cake, sprinkle with 2 teaspoons of the brown sugar crystals, and bake for about 1 hour, or until well risen and a toothpick inserted into the center comes out clean. Cool in the pan for 30 minutes, and turn out onto a wire rack to cool completely.

Make the cider crunch topping just before serving: mix the cider with the remaining brown sugar crystals to make a wet paste. Dot the crunchy paste over the cake.

☐ **TO STORE:** The cake will keep for 1 week, without the topping, in an airtight container.

✷ **TO FREEZE:** Wrap the cake, without the topping, in parchment paper and foil, and freeze in an airtight container. Defrost for 1–2 hours, and top with the crunchy cider topping after defrosting.

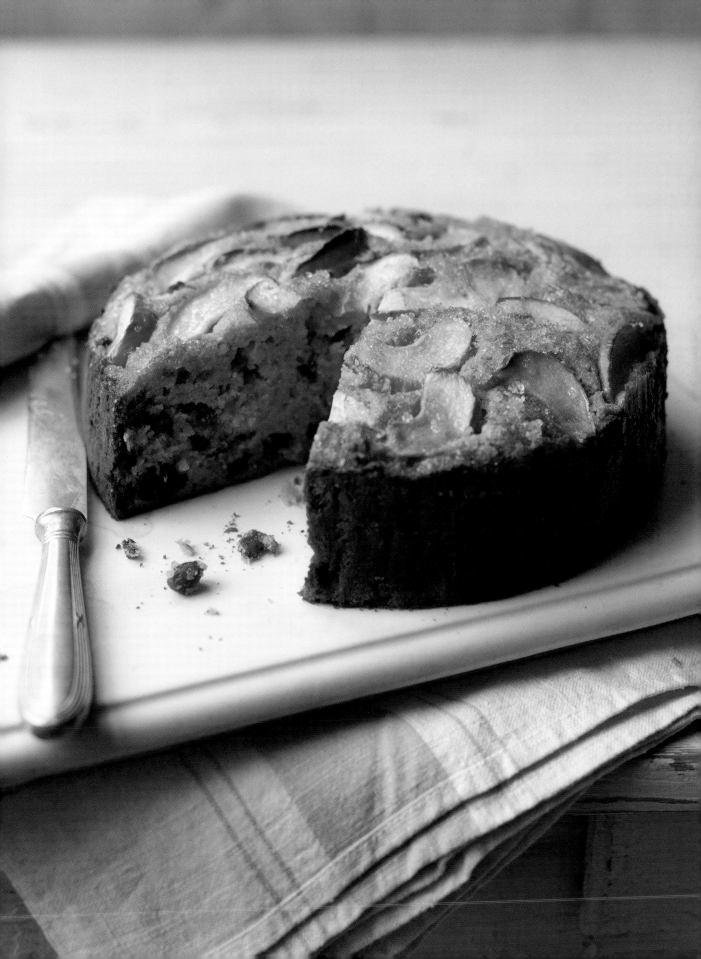

CHOCOLATE BROWNIE TORTE

Everybody likes chocolate brownies! This recipe is a variation and makes a really gooey and rich torte.

MAKES: ONE 8-INCH (20 CM) ROUND CAKE
PREPARATION: 20 MINUTES
BAKING: 30 MINUTES, PLUS 15 MINUTES COOLING

---

vegetable oil, for oiling

1²⁄₃ cups (10 oz) bittersweet chocolate (see box, page 19)

5 large eggs, separated, at room temperature

¾ cup (6 oz) superfine sugar

1¼ cups (5 oz) ground almonds

sifted confectioners' sugar, for dusting

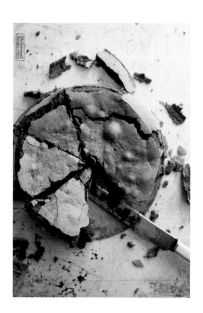

Preheat the oven to 325°F (160°C). Oil an 8-inch (20 cm) round cake pan with a removable bottom, and line base with parchment paper.

Roughly chop about ¹⁄₃ cup (2 oz) of the chocolate, and set aside. Melt the remaining chocolate, either in the microwave or in a heatproof bowl set over a pan of simmering water, and cool slightly.

Whisk the egg whites in a very clean bowl until they form soft peaks. Gradually whisk in half the sugar, a tablespoon at a time, until incorporated and you have a soft meringue.

Using a hand-held electric mixer, beat the egg yolks together with the remaining sugar in a large mixing bowl, until pale and doubled in volume. Carefully fold half the meringue mixture into the egg yolk mixture, so you keep all the air in. Gently fold in the melted chocolate, then carefully fold in the rest of the meringue mixture. Finally fold in the ground almonds and the chopped chocolate.

Spoon the mixture into the pan, level it, and bake in the center of the oven for 30 minutes. Turn the oven off, and leave the cake inside for 15 minutes—it will continue baking as the oven cools. Remove the cake from the oven, and leave to cool completely in the pan on a wire rack.

The surface of the torte will be cracked (the cracks are part of its charm) and crusted, and underneath it will be soft and moist. Dust the top with confectioners' sugar to serve.

Variation

If you like, you could add 2–3 tablespoons of orange liqueur when you add the melted chocolate to the cake mixture.

☐ **TO STORE:** The cake will keep for 3–4 days in an airtight container in the fridge.

✱ **TO FREEZE:** Wrap the undusted cake in parchment paper, and place it in an airtight container. Defrost for 1–2 hours, then dust with confectioners' sugar.

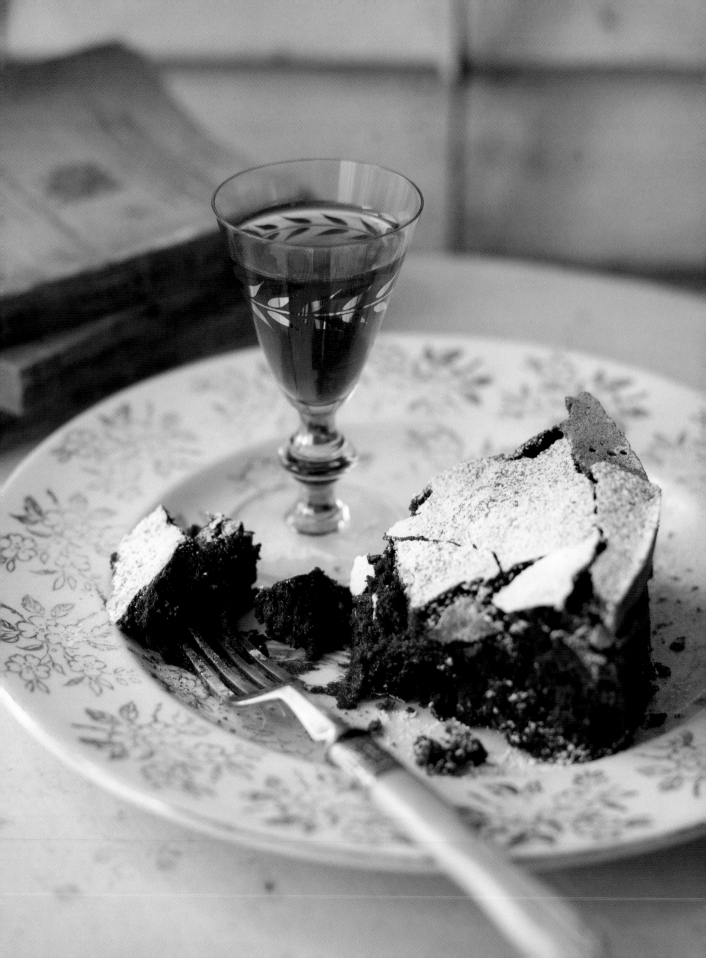

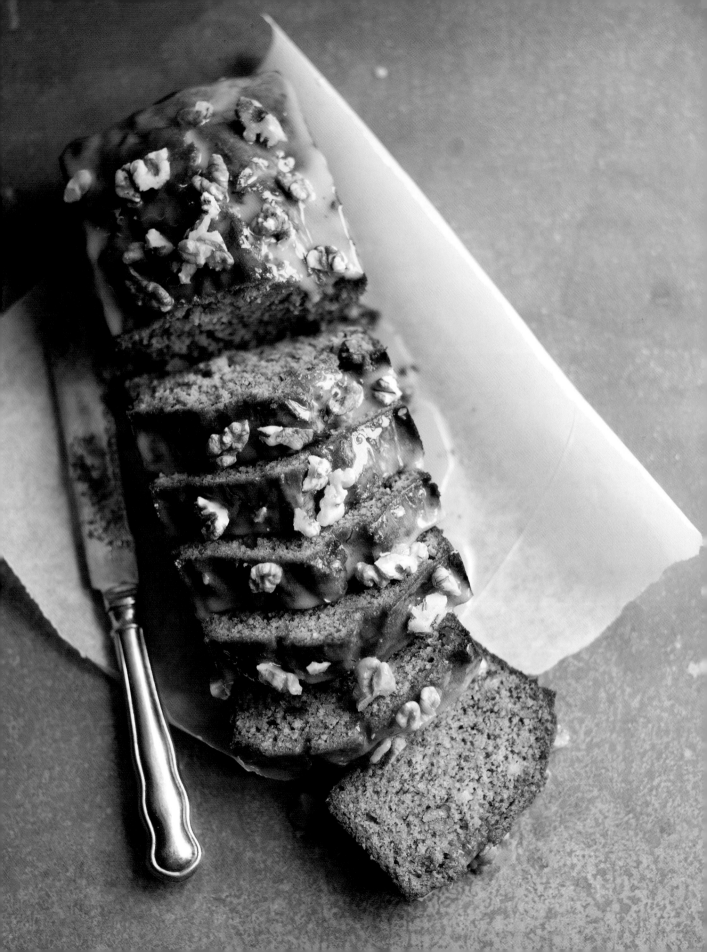

ROASTED BANANA WALNUT CAKE WITH MAPLE FROSTING

This combines some of my favorite flavors in one moist sponge cake. Made with roasted bananas for a great texture, and drizzled with deliciously sticky maple frosting—fantastic!

MAKES: ONE 9 × 5-INCH (23 × 13 CM, 2 LB) LOAF
PREPARATION: 15 MINUTES
BAKING: 40–50 MINUTES

For the cake

1 lb bananas in their skins

generous ⅔ cup (5 oz) light brown sugar

½ cup (4 fl oz) sunflower oil

1 teaspoon glycerin

3 large eggs, at room temperature

2 cups (8 oz) Gluten-Free Flour Mix B (see page 22)

½ teaspoon xanthan gum

½ teaspoon baking soda

½ teaspoon baking powder (see box, page 19)

2 tablespoons crème fraîche or sour cream

½ cup (2 oz) walnut pieces

For the maple frosting

3 tablespoons maple syrup

¾ cup (3 oz) fondant icing sugar (see page 40)

crushed walnuts, to decorate

Preheat the oven to 400°F (200°C).

Make a slit in each banana and place on a baking sheet. Roast the bananas in their skins for about 10 minutes, until soft. Cool, peel, mash roughly, and set aside.

Reduce oven temperature to 350°F (180°C). Oil a 9 × 5-inch (2 lb) loaf pan, and line base with parchment paper.

Tip the sugar into a large mixing bowl and, using a hand-held electric mixer, whisk in the oil, glycerin, and eggs, one at a time.

Sift together the flour, xanthan gum, baking soda, and baking powder, and mix this into the bowl, with the crème fraîche or sour cream. Stir in the mashed banana and the walnuts, and mix all the ingredients thoroughly.

Smooth the mixture in the prepared pan, and bake for about 45 minutes, until firm and springy when touched. Test with a toothpick, which should come out clean when inserted into the center. Cool in the pan for 10 minutes. Turn the cake out of the pan, peel off the paper, and cool on a wire rack.

For the icing, mix the maple syrup into the fondant icing sugar, with just enough water to make a runny icing. Set the cake on a serving plate, drizzle with the maple glaze, and scatter some crushed walnuts on top. Cut into slices to serve.

☐ **TO STORE:** The unfrosted cake will keep for 1 week in an airtight container.

✳ **TO FREEZE:** Wrap the unfrosted cake in parchment paper and foil, and freeze in an airtight container. Defrost for 1–2 hours, and frost after defrosting.

PLUM & ALMOND BUTTER CAKE

This is a buttery sponge cake with moist, sweet fruit to cut into wedges. Try it in autumn when plums are in season. Or, alternatively, choose cherries, peaches, nectarines, or apricots in the summer months.

This cake can be warmed before serving and enjoyed as a dessert with ice cream or served cold—and it's great for picnics.

MAKES: ONE 8-INCH (20 CM) ROUND CAKE
PREPARATION: 20 MINUTES
BAKING: 40–45 MINUTES

---

vegetable oil, for oiling

3 large eggs, at room temperature

2 teaspoons vanilla extract

generous ½ cup (4½ oz) superfine sugar

2 cups (7 oz) Gluten-Free Flour Mix B (see page 22)

1 tablespoon baking powder (see box, page 19)

1 teaspoon xanthan gum

½ cup (4 oz) unsalted butter, melted

1 teaspoon glycerin

3 tablespoons 2% milk

4-6 medium (12–14 oz) red plums, quartered and pitted

2 tablespoons light brown sugar

generous cup (4½ oz) slivered almonds

Preheat the oven to 350°F. Oil an 8-inch (20cm) round cake pan with a removable bottom, and line base with parchment paper.

Put the eggs into a bowl with the vanilla extract and superfine sugar. Using a hand-held electric mixer, whisk until light and the mixture forms a trail. Sift the flour with the baking powder and the xanthan gum, mix thoroughly, and fold into the mixture, stirring lightly, so you don't lose all the air in the batter. Stir in the melted butter, glycerin, and milk. Do not overbeat.

Put a layer of cake mixture in the pan. Scatter with some of the plums, then spoon in the rest of the cake batter. Tip the remaining plums on top. Sprinkle the light brown sugar and almonds over the fruit.

Place the cake on a baking sheet and bake for about 45 minutes, until the plums have begun to caramelize and a toothpick inserted into the center of the cake comes out clean. Remove the cake from the oven, leave to cool slightly, then gently loosen the sides. Transfer to a wire rack to cool completely.

☐ **TO STORE:** The cake will keep for 1 week in an airtight container.

✱ **TO FREEZE:** Wrap the cake in parchment paper and foil, and freeze in an airtight container.

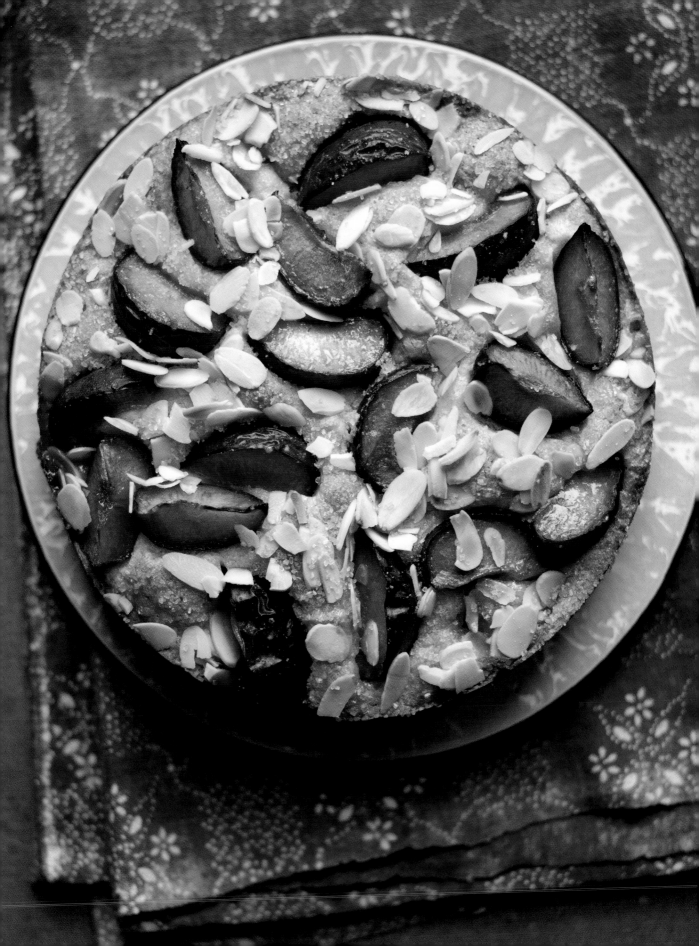

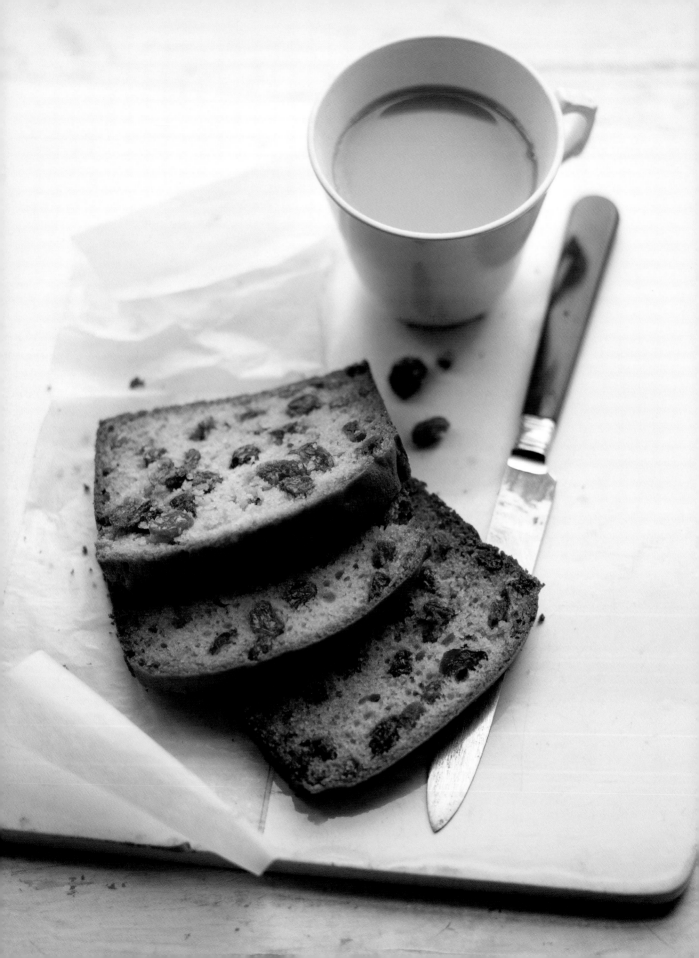

QUICK EXTRA MOIST FRUIT CAKE

One of the best pieces of advice I was ever given was to soak the fruit before making any fruit cake, and then taste the difference. It makes perfect sense if you think about it— dried fruit will reconstitute during cooking, drawing moisture from the baked sponge and making the cake dry. Soaking the fruit simply ensures you have a deliciously moist cake.

MAKES: ONE 9 × 5-INCH
   (23 × 13 CM, 2 LB) LOAF
PREPARATION: 15 MINUTES,
   PLUS 2 HOURS SOAKING TIME
BAKING: 50–60 MINUTES

½ cup (3½ oz) raisins

½ cup (3½ oz) golden raisins

½ cup (3 oz) dried cranberries

generous ½ cup (4½ fl oz) 2%
   milk, warmed

vegetable oil, for oiling

7 tablespoons (3¼ oz)
   margarine

generous ½ cup (4½ oz)
   superfine sugar

1¼ cups (6½oz) Gluten-Free
   Flour Mix A (see page 22)

1 teaspoon baking soda

1½ teaspoons baking powder
   (see box, page 19)

1 teaspoon xanthan gum

generous ½ cup (4½ fl oz)
   2% milk, warmed with
   2 teaspoons glycerin

2 large eggs, beaten,
   at room temperature

Place the fruit in a bowl, add the warmed milk, and stir well. Leave for at least 2 hours, or until the milk has been absorbed.

Preheat the oven to 325˚F. Oil a 9 × 5-inch (23 × 13 cm, 2 lb) loaf pan, and line base with parchment paper.

Place the margarine and sugar in a mixing bowl, and beat until nice and creamy. In a separate bowl, mix the flour, baking soda, baking powder, and xanthan gum really well. Add the flour mix to the margarine and sugar, then add the warm milk and glycerin, and mix well. Stir in the beaten eggs. Finally add the soaked fruit and liquid, and spoon into the prepared pan.

Bake in the oven for 50–60 minutes. The cake is ready when a toothpick inserted into the center of the cake comes out clean.

Once baked, remove from the oven, and cool for 5 minutes in the pan, then transfer to a wire rack to cool completely.

☐ **TO STORE:** The cake will keep for 1 week in an airtight container.

✱ **TO FREEZE:** Wrap well in plastic wrap, and freeze.

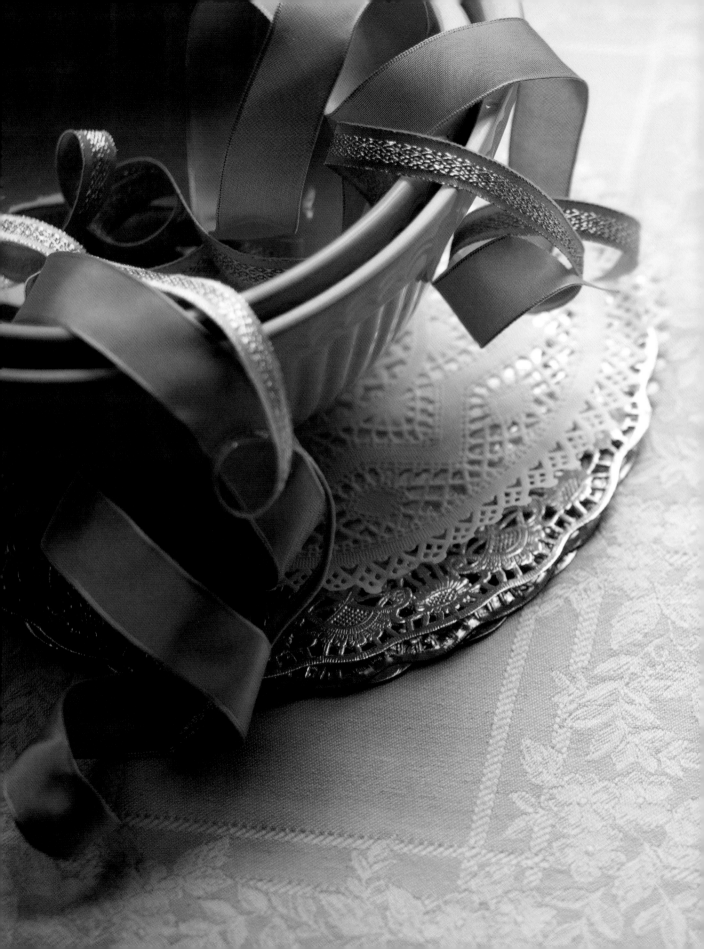

SPECIAL OCCASION CAKES

VANILLA & RASPBERRY CAKE

In my book *Seriously Good! Gluten-Free Cooking* there is a lovely birthday cake recipe. Since the publication of that book, I have had many inquiries about cakes for kids, so here is another version by special request.

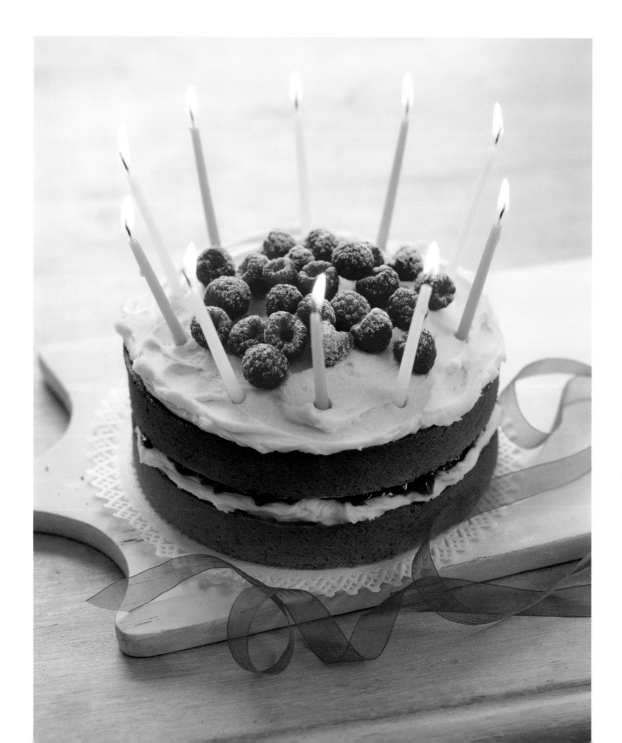

MAKES: ONE 8-INCH (20 CM) ROUND SPONGE CAKE
PREPARATION: 15 MINUTES, PLUS COOLING AND DECORATING
BAKING: 30 MINUTES

For the sponge cake

vegetable oil, for oiling

generous 1½ cups (12½ oz) superfine sugar

4 large eggs, at room temperature

2 teaspoons vanilla extract

2 teaspoons glycerin

3½ cups (12½ oz) Gluten-Free Flour Mix B (see page 22)

1 teaspoon xanthan gum

1 tablespoon baking powder (see box, page 19)

generous cup (8 fl oz) 2% milk

generous cup (8 fl oz) sunflower oil

For the buttercream frosting and decoration

1 cup (8 oz) unsalted butter, softened

4 cups (8 oz) confectioners' sugar, sifted

1 teaspoon vanilla extract

fresh raspberries

4 tablespoons raspberry jelly

edible glitter (see box, page 19)

Preheat the oven to 350°F (180°C). Oil two 8-inch (20 cm) layer cake pans and line base with parchment paper.

Place the superfine sugar, eggs, vanilla, and glycerin into a stand mixer, and whisk on high speed for 3 minutes. Sift together the flour, xanthan gum, and baking powder to combine evenly. In a measuring cup, mix the milk with the oil.

When the eggs are nice and thick, add the flour mixture. Return the bowl to the mixer, and slowly add the milk and the oil. Whisk thoroughly, but don't go mad.

Divide the mixture evenly between the pans, and level the surface. Bake on the same shelf in the center of the oven for 30–35, minutes until golden and firm. The cakes are ready when a toothpick inserted into the centers comes out clean.

Leave the cakes to cool in the pans for 15 minutes, and then turn out onto a wire rack to cool completely.

Peel off the lining paper, and decorate the cakes or freeze them (see below) until you are ready to use them.

To make the buttercream frosting, beat the butter with the confectioners' sugar and vanilla extract until light and fluffy.

Select the cake with the best-looking top, and set it aside. Turn the other cake over (trim the base to make it sit flat if necessary), and place it on a serving plate or cake board. Spread a layer of buttercream frosting over one cake, saving a generous amount for the top. Spread the same cake with raspberry jelly, and sandwich the two cakes together.

Spread the rest of the buttercream over the top of the cake. Top with fresh raspberries, and sprinkle with some edible glitter. The cake is best eaten on the same day that you frost and decorate it.

Filling variations
Buttercream frosting and jelly are a classic combination for filling a sponge cake, but you could also use lightly whipped cream with crushed fresh berries, or if the mood takes you, try lemon curd or marmalade and orange liqueur instead.

☐ **TO STORE:** The unfrosted cakes will keep for 2 days in an airtight container.

✱ **TO FREEZE:** Wrap the cooled cakes in plastic wrap, and store in the freezer for up to 3 months. Fill and frost the cake once it has defrosted.

GOOEY CHOCOLATE FUDGE CAKE

Everyone loves a chocolate cake. This light sponge, covered in shiny chocolate frosting, is superb. You would never know it was gluten-free!

MAKES: ONE 8-INCH (20 CM)
 ROUND CAKE
PREPARATION: 20 MINUTES,
 PLUS FILLING AND ICING
BAKING: 20–25 MINUTES

For the sponge cake

vegetable oil, for oiling

2 cups (8 oz) Gluten-Free Flour
 Mix B (see page 22)

1 teaspoon xanthan gum

1 teaspoon baking powder
 (see box, page 19)

½ teaspoon baking soda

½ cup (2 oz) cocoa powder

7½ tablespoons (3½ oz)
 unsalted butter, softened

1 cup (9 oz) dark brown sugar

3 large eggs, beaten, at
 room temperature

1 teaspoon vanilla extract

1 teaspoon glycerin

¾ cup (6½ fl oz) 2% milk

For the frosting

1¼ cups (8 oz) bittersweet
 chocolate (see box, page 19)

⅔ cup (5 fl oz) heavy whipping
 cream

7½ tablespoons (3½ oz)
 unsalted butter, softened

1 cup (4 oz) confectioners'
 sugar, sifted

Preheat the oven to 350°F (180°C). Oil two 8-inch (20 cm) layer cake pans and line base with parchment paper.

Sift the flour, xanthan gum, baking powder, baking soda, and cocoa powder together.

In a deep bowl, cream the butter and dark brown sugar together until light and fluffy. Gradually beat in the eggs, vanilla, and glycerin. Fold tablespoonfuls of the flour mixture into the butter and egg mixture, alternately with the milk, until the batter is evenly combined.

Divide the mixture between the pans, and level the surface. Bake on the same shelf in the center of the oven for about 25 minutes. The cakes are ready when a toothpick inserted into the center of the cakes comes out clean.

Leave the cakes to cool in the pans for 10 minutes, and then turn out onto a wire rack to cool completely.

For the frosting, melt the chocolate with the cream in a heatproof bowl in a microwave, or set over a pan of just simmering water. Stir very gently until the mixture is smooth. Allow to cool to room temperature. Cream the softened butter with the confectioners' sugar, and then beat this into the chocolate mixture until it is the consistency of soft butter.

Put one cake (top down) onto a serving plate and spread with some of the frosting, leaving a generous amount to completely cover the cakes. Sandwich with the second cake, and spread the rest of the frosting over the top and sides. Chill well in the fridge. Remove from the fridge 15 minutes before eating. Decorate with rose petals, silver leaf, or other decoration of your choice.

☐ **TO STORE:** The filled and frosted cake will keep for up to 3 days in an airtight container in the fridge.

✱ **TO FREEZE:** Freeze the frosted cake, uncovered. Once the frosting is set, cover, wrap well, and return to the freezer.

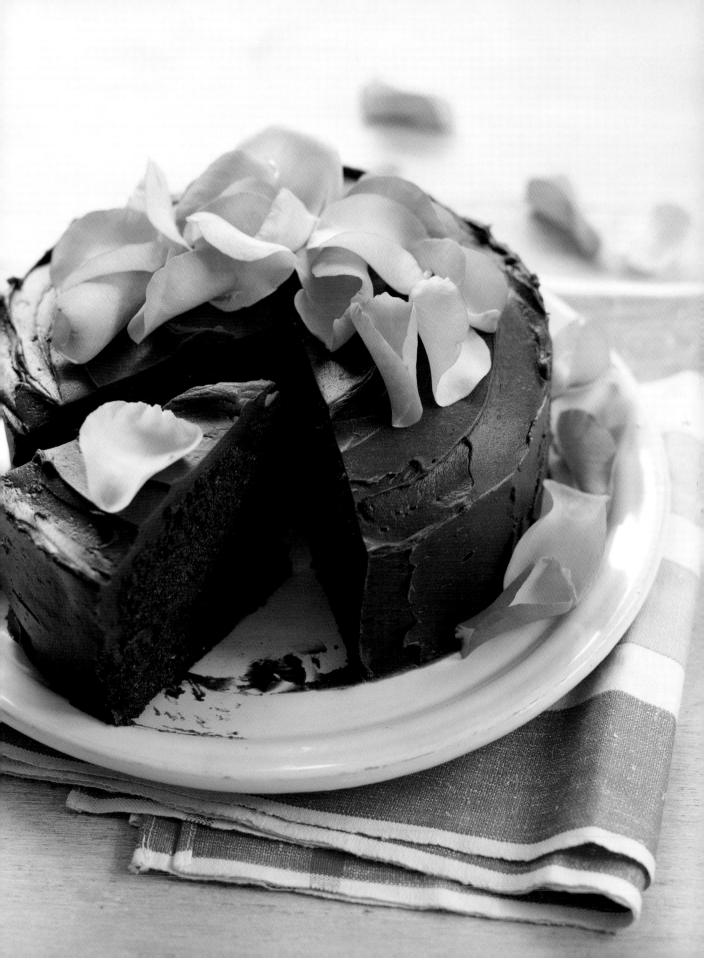

SIMNEL CAKE

This is a golden, rich British fruit cake topped with marzipan and traditionally served at Easter. It would also make a wonderful birthday or other special occasion cake.

MAKES: ONE 8-INCH (20 CM) ROUND CAKE
PREPARATION: 30 MINUTES
BAKING: 1½–1¾ HOURS

---

vegetable oil, for oiling

1 lb 2 oz marzipan (almond paste) (see box, page 19)

2 cups (8 oz) Gluten-Free Flour Mix B (see page 22)

1 teaspoon baking powder (see box, page 19)

1 teaspoon xanthan gum

½ teaspoon ground cinnamon

½ teaspoon ground allspice

½ teaspoon grated nutmeg

1 cup (8 oz) unsalted butter, softened

1 cup (8 oz) superfine sugar

4 large eggs, at room temperature

¼ cup (1 oz) ground almonds

2 tablespoons brandy

1¼ cups (8 oz) golden raisins

⅔ cup (4½ oz) currants

scant ½ cup (3½ oz) candied cherries, halved and washed

grated zest of 1 large lemon

For the top

2 tablespoons apricot jelly, warmed

4 tablespoons confectioners' sugar

2 teaspoons lemon juice

Preheat the oven to 325°F (160°C). Oil and line the base and sides of a 2½-inch (6 cm) deep, 8-inch (20 cm) round cake pan with a removable bottom with a double layer of parchment paper. Cut about 3 oz off the marzipan and set aside. Cut the remaining marzipan block in half.

Sift the flour, baking powder, xanthan gum, and spices together. In another bowl, beat the butter and the sugar together using a hand-held mixer, until fluffy and light.

Gradually add the eggs and the flour mixture alternately to the creamed mixture. Next, stir in the ground almonds. Stir in the brandy, then mix in the dried fruit, cherries, and lemon zest, and give the whole mixture a really good stir.

Spoon half of the batter into the pan, and level. Roll out one of the larger pieces of marzipan (use the base of the cake pan as a guide), and cut into a circle to fit the pan. Lay this carefully over the cake batter in the pan. Spoon in the remaining batter, level, and bake for 1½–1¾ hours, or until a toothpick inserted into the center of the cake comes out clean.

Leave the cake to cool in the pan. When it has cooled completely, take it out of the pan, remove the paper, and turn it upside down onto a serving plate, so you have a flat top.

Brush what is now the top of the cake with a little of the warmed apricot jelly. Roll out the larger remaining piece of marzipan to fit the top of the cake exactly and press it down flat. Flute the edges of the marzipan by "pinching" it.

Divide the reserved 3 oz of marzipan into 11 balls. Using the remaining jelly, stick the balls around the edges of the cake. Finally, mix a little lemon juice into the confectioners' sugar to give a soft spreading consistency, and pour it onto the center of the cake. Finish with a large ribbon around the side of the cake.

☐ **TO STORE:** Keeps for up to 1 week in an airtight container.

✱ **TO FREEZE:** Wrap the undecorated cake well in plastic wrap and foil, and freeze in an airtight container. Decorate with the marzipan once defrosted.

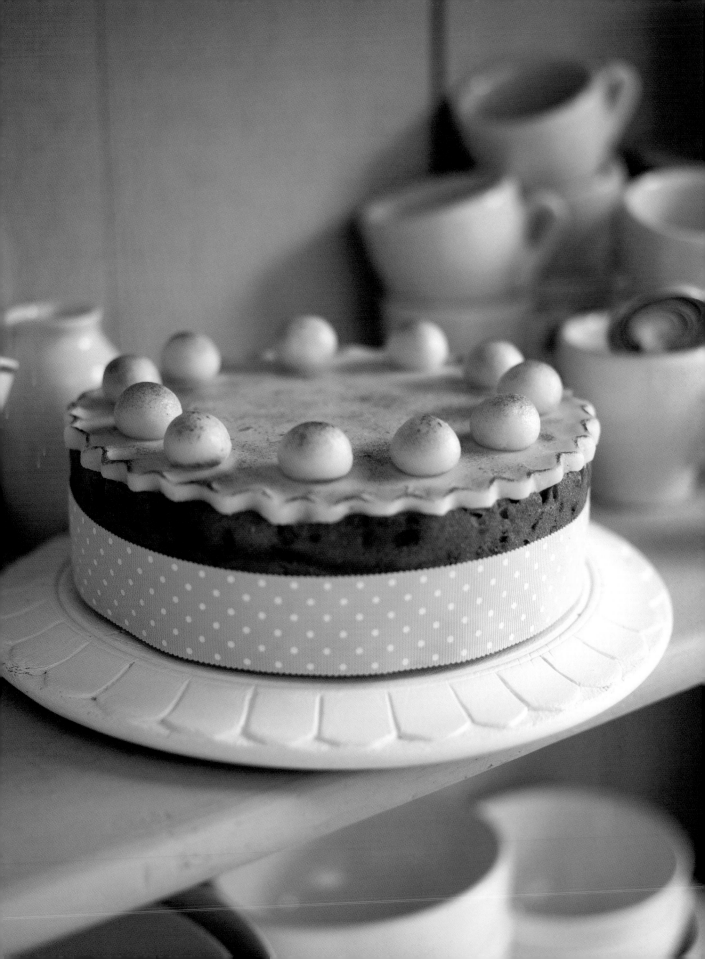

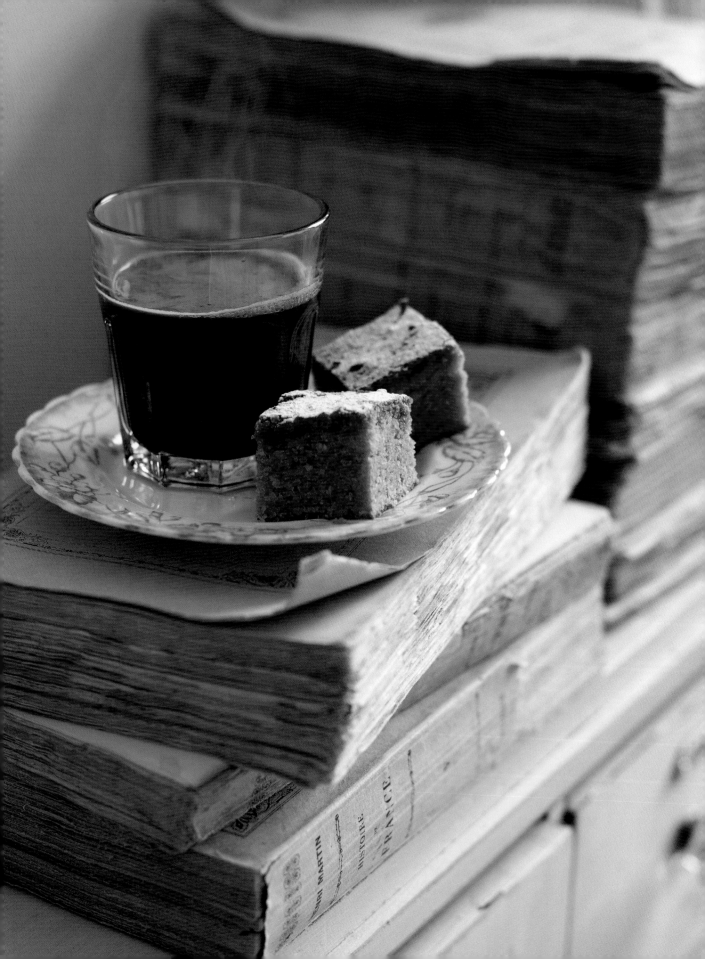

RICOTTA CAKE WITH COFFEE SYRUP

A few years ago I worked in northern Italy, where we would have a cake like this with coffee after lunch. The ricotta gives the cake a good texture and flavor, and the coffee syrup soaks in really well to finish it off perfectly. This is a great one for Father's Day!

MAKES: ONE 9-INCH (23 CM) SQUARE CAKE
PREPARATION: 15 MINUTES
BAKING: 35–40 MINUTES

For the cake

vegetable oil, for oiling

½ cup (4½ oz) unsalted butter, softened

generous ¾ cup (6½ oz) superfine sugar

⅔ cup (5 oz) ricotta cheese

2 large eggs, beaten, at room temperature

1¾ cups (7 oz) Gluten-Free Flour Mix B (see page 22)

2 teaspoons baking powder (see box, page 19)

1 teaspoon xanthan gum

2 teaspoons instant coffee dissolved in 2 tablespoons boiling water

For the syrup

½ cup (4 fl oz) brandy

½ cup (4 oz) superfine sugar

4 teaspoons instant coffee

sifted confectioners' sugar, for dusting

Preheat the oven to 350°F (180°C). Oil a 9-inch (23 cm) square cake pan, and line base with parchment paper.

Place the softened butter and sugar in a mixing bowl, and beat with a hand-held electric mixer until creamed together. Add the ricotta cheese and eggs, and mix well.

Next, sift the flour, baking powder, and xanthan gum together so that they are evenly mixed. Add this to the ricotta mixture, and finally stir in the coffee liquid. Mix well.

Spread into the prepared pan, and bake for about 35 minutes. The cake is ready when a toothpick inserted into the center of the cake comes out clean.

For the syrup, place the brandy, sugar, and coffee together into a saucepan, and bring to a simmer to dissolve the sugar. Turn the heat down and cook for 2 minutes to reduce. Set aside.

Once the cake is baked, remove it from the oven, cool slightly in the pan, and prick all over with a skewer. Pour over the warm syrup and leave to cool.

Once cooled, remove the cake from the pan, and peel off the paper. To serve, cut into squares, and dust with confectioners' sugar.

☐ **TO STORE:** The cake will keep for up to 1 week in an airtight container.

✳ **TO FREEZE:** Place the undusted cake in an airtight container, and freeze. Defrost for 1–2 hours, and when defrosted, sprinkle with confectioners' sugar.

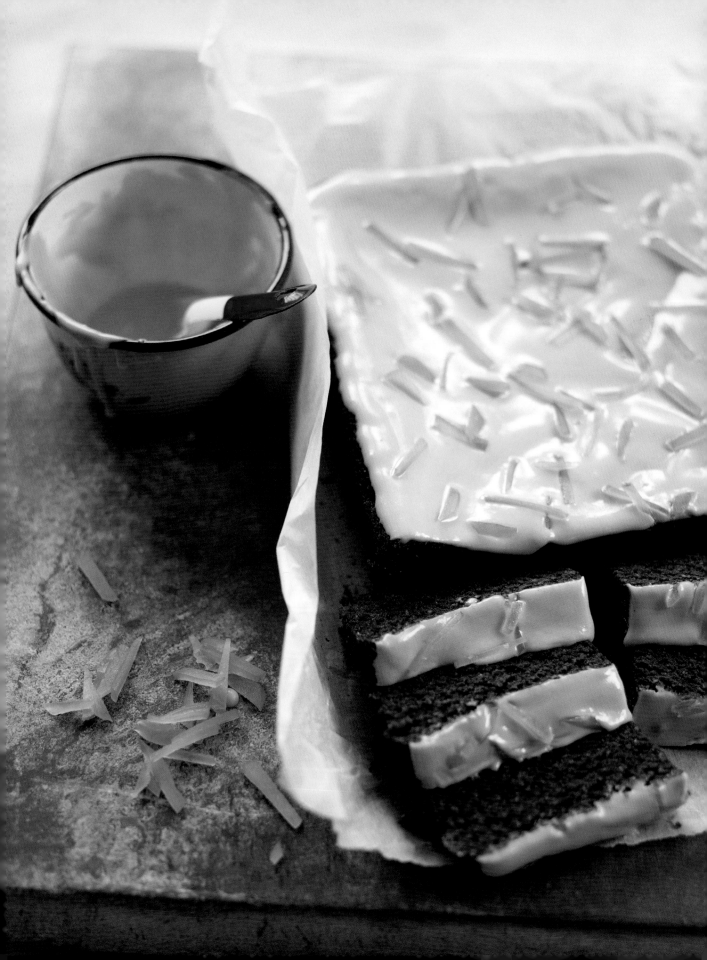

BONFIRE PARKIN WITH GINGER FROSTING

Parkin is a traditional ginger, molasses, and oat cake from Lancashire and Yorkshire, but this one is adapted from my mom's recipe—she always used to make it on Bonfire Night, celebrated in England on the 5th of November.

MAKES: ONE 9-INCH (23 CM) SQUARE CAKE
PREPARATION: 15 MINUTES
BAKING: 45 MINUTES

For the parkin

vegetable oil, for oiling

2 cups (8 oz) Gluten-Free Flour Mix B (see page 22)

1 teaspoon ground ginger

1 teaspoon pumpkin pie spice

1 teaspoon xanthan gum

2 cups (8 oz) very fine oatmeal (see box, page 19)

1⅔ cups (10 oz) molasses

1 cup (8 oz) superfine sugar

¾ cup (6 oz) unsalted butter, softened

1 teaspoon baking soda

generous ½ cup (4 fl oz) 2% milk

For the ginger icing

1⅓ cups (5½ oz) confectioners' sugar, sifted

2 tablespoons ginger syrup (from a jar of stem ginger)

few slivers of stem ginger, chopped

Preheat the oven to 350°F (180°C). Oil and line the base of a 9-inch (23 cm) square baking pan.

Sift the flour, ginger, pumpkin pie spice, and xanthan gum together. Add the oatmeal, and stir well. Gently heat the molasses, sugar, and butter together in a pan until melted, and nice and runny. Dissolve the baking soda in the milk. Pour the melted butter mixture into the dry ingredients, then add the milk mixture. Carefully stir together, and pour into the prepared baking pan.

Bake for about 45 minutes, or until well risen and firm. Allow the parkin to cool in the pan.

To make the icing, sift the confectioners' sugar into a bowl; add the ginger syrup, and just enough cold water to mix until smooth and thick. Spread the icing over the cooled cake, decorate with slivers of chopped stem ginger, then cut into slices.

☐ **TO STORE:** The cake will keep for 2 days stored in an airtight container.

✱ **TO FREEZE:** Wrap the unfrosted cake in parchment paper and foil, and freeze in an airtight container. Defrost for 1–2 hours, and when defrosted, frost and decorate as above.

RICH FRUIT CHRISTMAS CAKE

I actually prefer this gluten-free version of Christmas cake to the traditional kind. The texture is just the same if not better, and it is delicious! It's best to soak the fruit in the whiskey and lemon juice overnight; it makes a real difference to the texture of the cake.

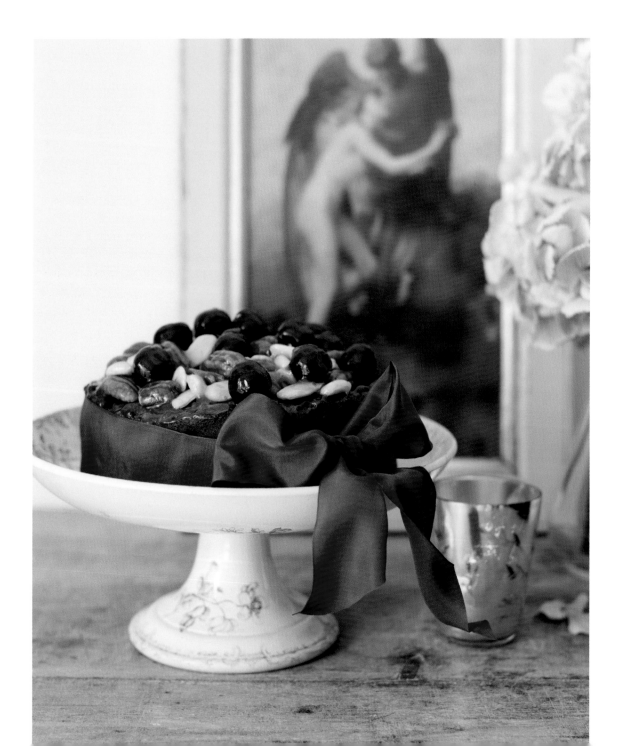

For the cake

½ cup (3 oz) currants

½ cup (3 oz) golden raisins

2 cups (13 oz) raisins

½ cup (2 oz) candied citrus peel

⅔ cup (5 fl oz) whiskey

grated zest and juice of
1 small lemon

vegetable oil, for oiling

1¼ cups (5¼ oz) Gluten-Free
Flour Mix B (see page 22)

1 teaspoon baking powder
(see box, page 19)

1 teaspoon xanthan gum

1 teaspoon pumpkin pie spice

1 teaspoon ground allspice

⅔ cup (5 oz) unsalted butter,
softened

⅔ cup (5 oz) soft dark brown
sugar

3 large eggs, at room
temperature

½ cup (2 oz) ground almonds

2 tablespoons 2% milk

½ cup whole almonds

scant ½ cup (3½ oz) candied
cherries, halved and washed

1 tablespoon molasses

1 tablespoon clear honey

For the top

2 tablespoons smooth apricot
jelly, warmed

½ cup (3½ oz) mixed candied
fruits, e.g., cherries, ginger,
melon or pineapple

½ cup (2 oz) nuts, e.g.,
almonds, walnuts, pecans

MAKES: ONE DEEP 7-INCH (18 CM)
ROUND OR SQUARE CAKE
PREPARATION: 20 MINUTES,
PLUS OVERNIGHT SOAKING TIME
BAKING: 1½–2 HOURS

Place the dried fruit and candied peel in a pan, add the whiskey, and the lemon juice and zest, and bring to a boil. Take the pan off the heat, cover, and leave to soak overnight.

Preheat the oven to 300°F (150°C). Oil and line the base of a 2½–3-inch (6–7.5 cm) deep round or square 7-inch (18 cm) cake pan, plus a tall collar overlapped around the sides, with a double layer of parchment paper.

Sift the flour, baking powder, xanthan gum, and spices together. Cream the butter and sugar together until fluffy and light. Gradually add the eggs and flour alternately, and then add the ground almonds. Stir in the milk, and mix in the dried fruit mixture, almonds, and cherries. Finally stir in the molasses and honey, and give the whole cake mixture a thoroughly good stir.

Spoon the mixture into the pan, level, and bake for about 1½–2 hours, or until a toothpick inserted into the center comes out clean. Leave to cool in the pan.

To decorate, brush the surface of the cake with half the warmed jelly. Arrange or pile a selection of candied fruits and nuts over the top, and brush with another layer of jelly to glaze. Now all you need is a big bow to put around the sides!

Prefer a traditional topping?

I like the candied fruit and nut topping as it's so quick and easy! But if you prefer, decorate it in the traditional way with a layer of marzipan topped with frosting of your choice.

☐ **TO STORE:** The undecorated cake will keep for up to 1 month, tightly wrapped in foil in an airtight container.

✻ **TO FREEZE:** When cold, remove the cake from the pan, wrap in parchment paper and two thick layers of foil, and freeze in an airtight container. Defrost for 3–4 hours, and when defrosted, decorate as above.

CHOCOLATE CHERRY TRIFLE CAKE

MAKES: ONE TALL 8-INCH
  (20 CM) CAKE
PREPARATION: 20 MINUTES
BAKING: 12–15 MINUTES

---

vegetable oil, for oiling

2 large eggs, at room
  temperature

1 cup (8 oz) superfine sugar

1¼ cups (6¼ oz) Gluten-Free
  Flour Mix A (see page 22)

pinch of salt

1½ teaspoons baking powder
  (see box, page 19)

1 teaspoon xanthan gum

3 tablespoons cocoa powder,
  sifted

½ cup (4 fl oz) sunflower oil

½ cup (4 fl oz) 2% milk

2 teaspoons vanilla extract

1 teaspoon glycerin, optional

For the filling

⅔ cup (3 oz) instant custard
  powder (see box, page 19)

scant cup (5½ oz) bittersweet
  chocolate (see box, page 19),
  finely chopped

scant cup (5½ oz) white
  chocolate (see box, page 19),
  finely chopped

2½ cups (20 fl oz) heavy cream

3 tablespoons confectioners'
  sugar

15 oz can cherries in syrup,
  drained well

This cake is great at Christmas when you want something different from the usual. The glycerin is an optional extra and helps to give the cake a little more shelf life.

Preheat the oven to 350°F (180°C). Oil two 8-inch (20 cm) layer cake pans.

Whisk the eggs and sugar together in a medium bowl for about 1 minute by hand. In a separate bowl, mix the flour, salt, baking powder, xanthan gum, and cocoa powder together really well. Whisk the oil, milk, vanilla, and glycerin together in a bowl. Add the dry ingredients to the beaten eggs and sugar, then mix in the wet ingredients.

Divide the mixture evenly between the oiled pans, and bake for 12–15 minutes, or until well risen and spongy when pressed lightly in the center. Leave to cool.

Divide the instant custard powder equally between two clean bowls, and then pour ⅔ cup (5 fl oz) boiling water into each bowl, whisking well. Add the white chocolate to one bowl and the bittersweet chocolate to the other, whisking well to melt the chocolate completely. Then set aside to cool until thickened.

Lightly whip the cream with the confectioners' sugar.

Carefully slice each cooled cake in half widthwise. Place one sponge layer on a serving plate. Spread some bittersweet chocolate custard onto it, then dot with some cherries and fill in the gaps with a little white chocolate custard and whipped cream. Continue layering the sponges and fillings in this way until you reach the top (make sure you save enough whipped cream for the topping). Press the final sponge down lightly.

Spread whipped cream over the top of the cake, and decorate with some canned or fresh cherries. Scatter with some chocolate sprinkles for that finishing touch.

☐ **TO STORE:** The decorated cakes will keep for 1 day in an airtight container.

✳ **TO FREEZE:** The plain sponges can be frozen. Wrap in foil, and freeze in an airtight container. Defrost for 1–2 hours.

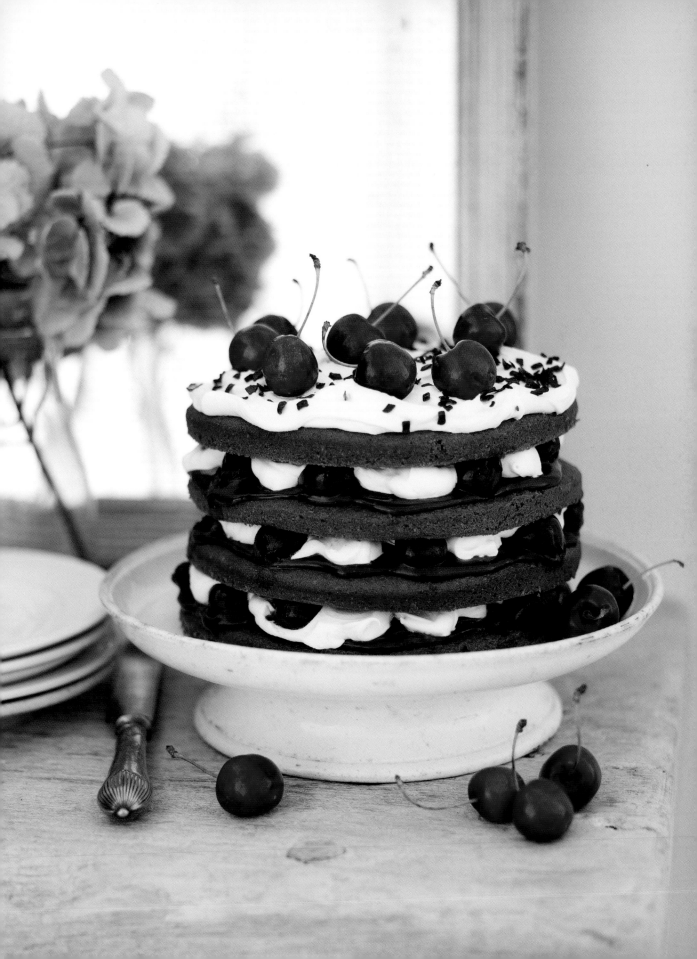

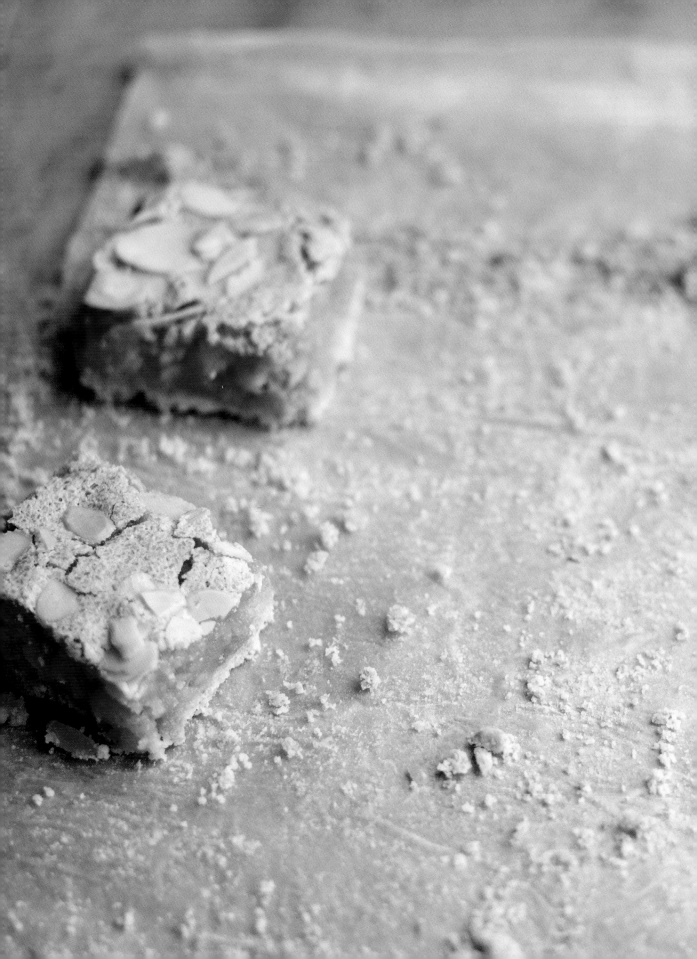

SHEET CAKES & BARS

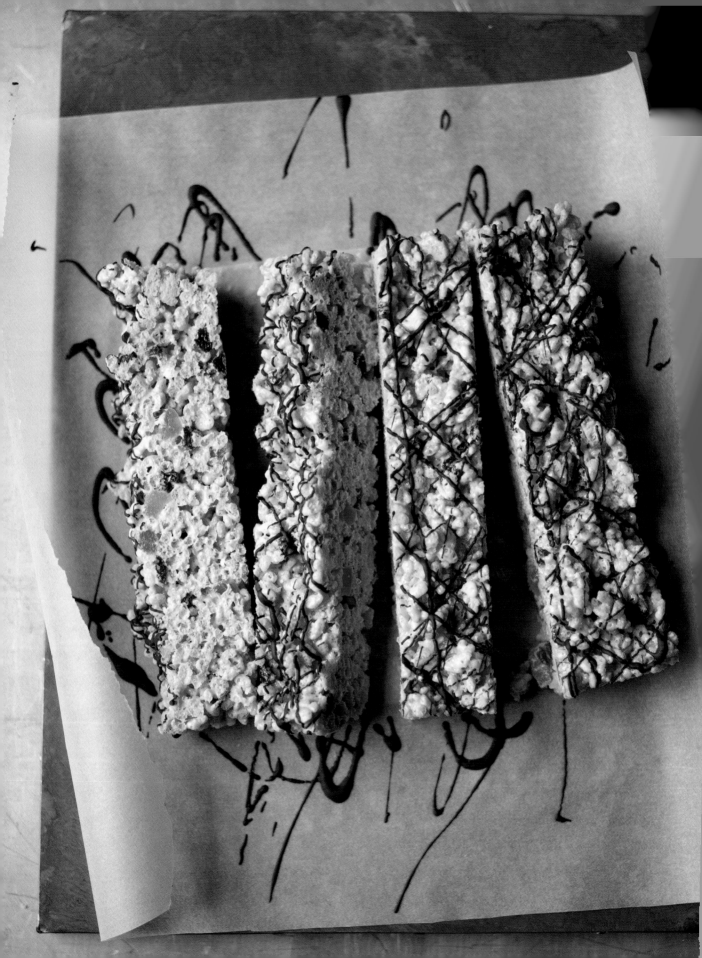

MARSHMALLOW CRISPIES

Classic kids' stuff here, but I have seen many an adult tuck into these at a kids' party … be warned, they are very addictive!

MAKES: 16 BARS
PREPARATION: 10 MINUTES
BAKING: 10 MINUTES

---

vegetable oil, for oiling

¼ cup (2 oz) unsalted butter

29 marshmallows (7 oz)
   (see box, page 19)

scant cup (5¼ oz) mixed dried
   fruit, e.g., chopped apricots
   and raisins

2 gluten-free cookies (2 oz) or
   shortbread (try the recipe on
   page 23), crumbled

4½ cups (5 oz) gluten-free crisp
   puffed rice cereal

½ cup (3 oz) bittersweet
   chocolate (see box, page 19)

Oil a 9½-inch (24 cm) square baking pan and line base with parchment paper.

Melt the butter in a medium nonstick pan. Next add the marshmallows, and stir over low heat until completely melted; take care not to burn or boil the mixture. Off the heat, stir in the fruit, the crumbled cookies, and finally add the crisp puffed rice cereal. Mix well.

Press the mixture down lightly into the prepared pan.

Melt the chocolate in a heatproof bowl in a microwave, or set over a pan of just simmering water—don't let the bowl touch the water. Drizzle the chocolate over the cake and leave to chill in the fridge until firm.

Cut into 16 rectangles or squares to serve.

☐ **TO STORE:** The crispies will keep for 1 week stored in an airtight container.

✴ **TO FREEZE:** Wrap well, and freeze in a plastic bag.

PECAN HONEY OAT BARS

This recipe is bulked up with the addition of roasted pecans. They really add to the flavor and texture.

MAKES: 10–12 BARS
PREPARATION: 10 MINUTES
BAKING: 15–20 MINUTES

---

vegetable oil, for oiling

scant cup (3½ oz) pecan halves, roughly chopped

very scant cup (7 oz) unsalted butter

scant cup (7 oz) dark brown sugar

⅔ cup (7 oz) clear honey

4⅔ cups (14 oz) rolled oats (see box, page 19)

⅔ cup (3½ oz) sesame seeds

1⅓ cups (6 oz) dried cranberries

2 teaspoons ground allspice

Preheat the oven to 350°F (180°C). Line a baking sheet with parchment paper. Oil a 13 × 9-inch (33 × 23 cm) baking pan, and line base with parchment paper.

Place the pecans on the lined sheet, and toast them well in the oven for 8–10 minutes. Once browned, remove from the oven and cool.

Increase the oven temperature to 400°F (200°C).

Melt the butter in a medium nonstick pan. Then add the sugar and honey, and mix well until the sugar has dissolved. Add the pecans, oats, sesame seeds, cranberries, and allspice, and mix really well. Spoon the mixture into the prepared baking pan, and press down evenly.

Bake for 15–20 minutes, or until golden.

Once baked, allow the oat bars to cool in the pan, then cut into 10–12 even pieces.

☐ **TO STORE:** The oat bars will keep for 1 week in an airtight container.

✱ **TO FREEZE:** Wrap well, and store in a plastic bag.

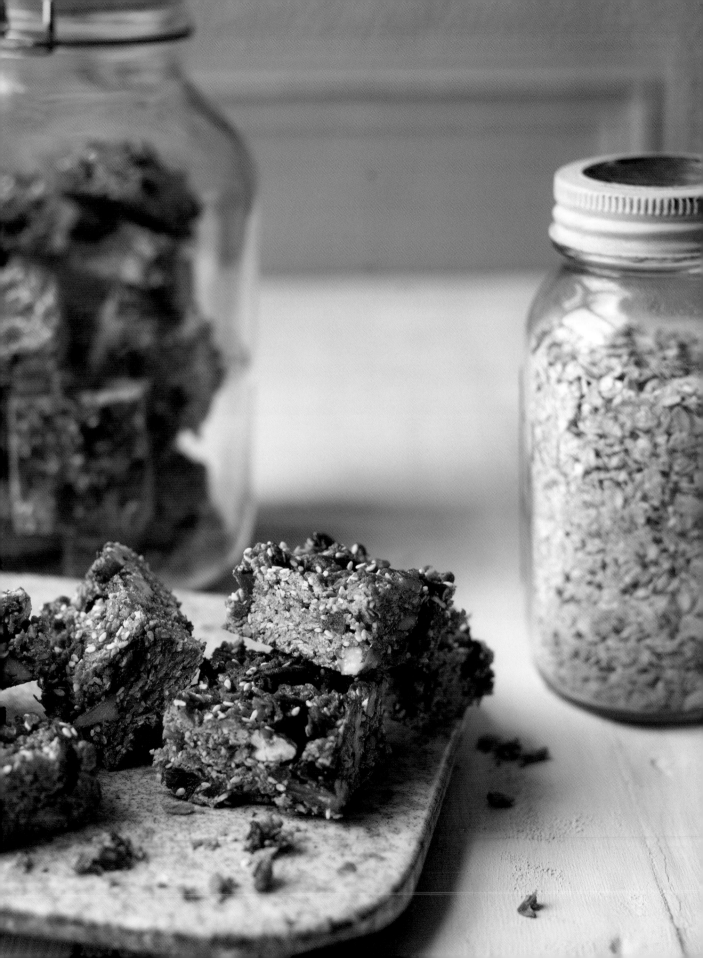

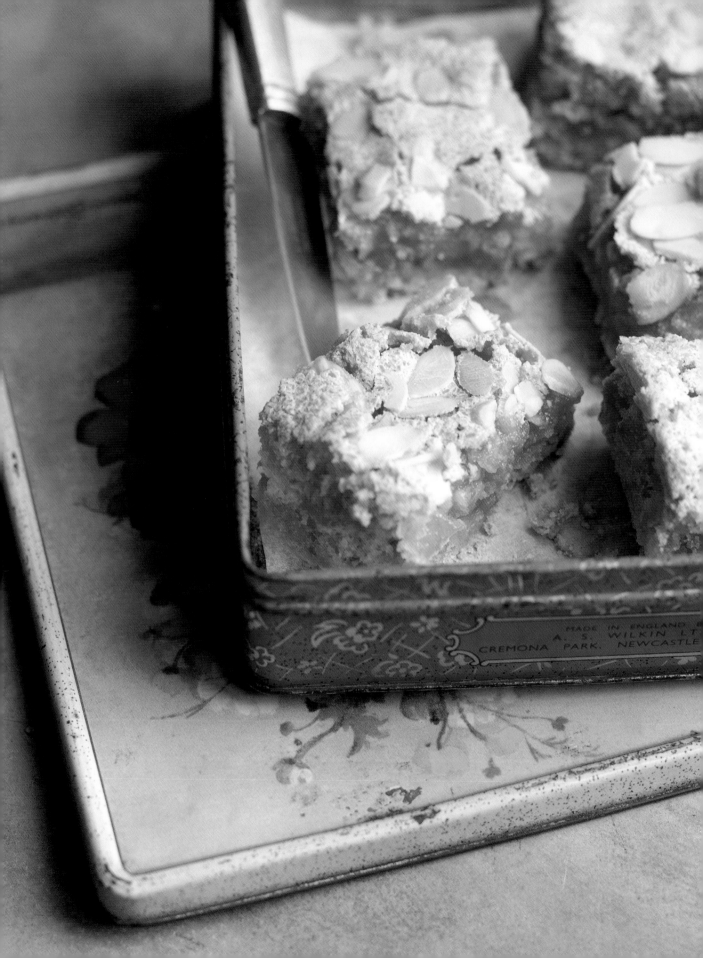

APRICOT & ALMOND MACAROON BARS

These have a lovely chewy texture and make a really tasty treat for a picnic or lunch box.

MAKES: 16 BARS
PREPARATION: 20 MINUTES
BAKING: 40–45 MINUTES

For the base

vegetable oil, for oiling

1⅛ cups (5¼ oz) rice flour

¼ cup (2 oz) superfine sugar

2 tablespoons (1 oz) dark brown sugar

6 tablespoons (3 oz) unsalted butter, cubed

4 tablespoons apricot jelly

For the filling/topping

1¼ cups (8 oz) soft dried apricots, roughly chopped

1 tablespoon lemon juice

2 large eggs, at room temperature

1 teaspoon vanilla extract

generous ½ cup (4½ oz) light brown sugar

3 tablespoons rice flour

½ teaspoon baking powder (see box, page 19)

½ cup (2 oz) ground almonds

light brown sugar and sliced almonds, for sprinkling

Preheat the oven to 350°F (180°C). Oil a 9-inch (23 cm) square baking pan, and line base with parchment paper.

Put the flour and sugars for the base into a food processor, and blend together. Add the butter, and process until the mixture forms fine crumbs, and then starts to clump together. Tip the crumb mixture into the base of the prepared pan, and press lightly to make an even layer.

Bake the base for 10–15 minutes, or until pale golden brown. When cool, brush with the apricot jelly.

Meanwhile, put the apricots into a small pan with the lemon juice and 5 tablespoons cold water. Stir over low heat until soft, thick, and fairly smooth. Cool slightly, then spread over the base and set aside.

Start whisking the eggs and the vanilla together, then whisk in the sugar until thickened and airy. Stir the flour and baking powder together, and fold into the sugar-egg mixture. Finally, fold in the ground almonds.

Spoon the topping onto the apricot layer and sprinkle the light brown sugar and sliced almonds on top. Return the pan to the oven for about 30 minutes, until golden and risen.

Remove from the oven and allow to cool in the pan, then cut into 16 bars.

☐ **TO STORE:** The bars will keep for 1 week stored in an airtight container.

✳ **TO FREEZE:** Wrap well, and freeze in an airtight container.

FUDGY COFFEE MACADAMIA CRUNCH

This is a really tasty sweet treat, but take care not to overbeat the egg whites, or the texture will end up slightly firmer than desired. I like to add alternate spoonfuls of the two mixtures to the pan to give a nice marbled effect.

Any nuts will do for the praline topping, or you can just use the sugar on its own.

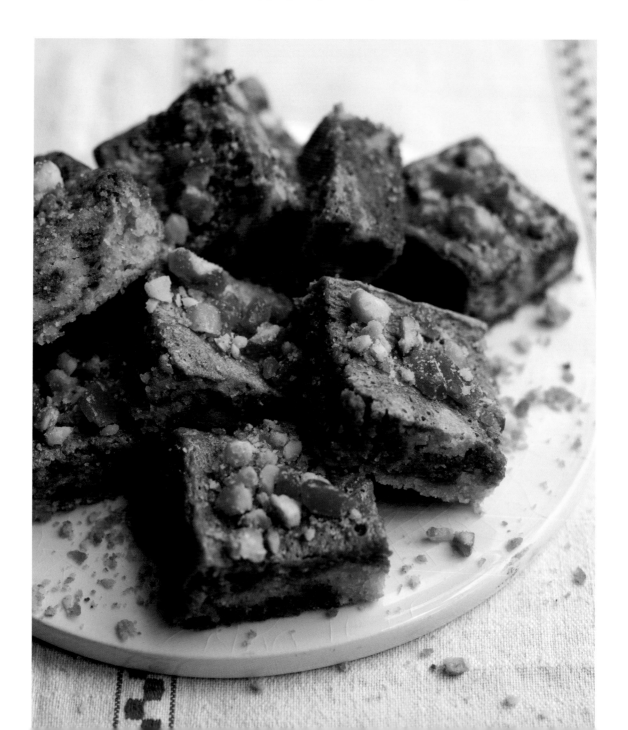

MAKES: 9 SQUARES
PREPARATION: 25 MINUTES
BAKING: 30 MINUTES

For the sponge base

vegetable oil, for oiling

¾ cup (6 oz) unsalted butter

5 extra large eggs, separated,
   at room temperature

scant cup (7 oz) soft light brown
   sugar

1¾ cups (7 oz) ground almonds
   (see Cook's note, below)

1 teaspoon xanthan gum

2 tablespoons instant coffee
   dissolved in 1 tablespoon
   boiling water

For the praline topping

½ cup (3½ oz) superfine sugar

¾ cup (3½ oz) macadamia nuts

Cook's note

For the sponge base, I like to
use whole blanched almonds,
and grind them myself, either
in a food processor or by
bashing them in a sealed bag
with a rolling pin. This gives
a slightly different texture, and
I think it tastes even better.

Preheat the oven to 350°F (180°C). Oil a 9-inch (23 cm) square
baking pan, and line base with parchment paper. Oil or line
a baking sheet with parchment paper for the praline.

Melt the butter in a small pan. Stir the egg yolks into
the sugar in a large mixing bowl, then gradually add the
melted butter.

Whisk the egg whites until they form soft peaks. Fold the
whites into the yolk mixture very lightly, so you don't lose
all the air, and then add the ground almonds and the xanthan
gum, very gently. Put half the mixture into a separate bowl,
and mix the coffee liquid into that portion.

Spoon some of each mixture alternately into the prepared
pan, and repeat to create layers; drag a spoon back and forth
a couple of times to create a marbled mixture.

Bake in the center of the oven for about 30 minutes. The
top will be firm, and the center still a bit soft. Stand the pan
on a wire rack, and leave to cool completely.

To make the praline topping, place the sugar and macadamia
nuts together in a large skillet over low heat. Keep
watching; swirl the pan occasionally, until all the sugar has
completely dissolved to a rich brown liquid (about 10 minutes).
You may have to stir the last of the sugar crystals in, and
keep an eye on the pan, because it burns easily.

Pour this mixture onto the prepared baking sheet, spreading
the macadamia nuts out in a single layer. Leave the mixture
to cool and become brittle, then lift it off the baking sheet
into a double-layer strong freezer bag. Break it up with a
few bashes from a rolling pin, and then crush it quite finely
with the rolling pin.

Remove the cake from the pan, and peel off the paper. Turn
it right side up, and place on a board, then spoon the praline
on top of the cake, and cut into squares.

☐ **TO STORE:** The bars will keep for 1 week stored in an
   airtight container.

✻ **TO FREEZE:** Cool the sponge, wrap well, and freeze,
   without the topping. Add the praline topping after defrosting.

CHOCOLATE CARAMEL ROCKY ROAD SHORTBREAD

I just had to put this in the book! It is fast becoming a real classic; everywhere you go these days, rocky road is on the menu. Cutting it into thick squares is the only option here.

MAKES: 12 LARGE SQUARES
PREPARATION: 15 MINUTES,
    PLUS CHILLING AND SETTING
BAKING: 15–20 MINUTES

___

For the base

vegetable oil, for oiling

¾ cup (3½ oz) cornstarch

¾ cup (3½ oz) rice flour

¼ cup (2 oz) superfine sugar

2 tablespoons dark brown sugar

½ cup (4 oz) unsalted butter, cubed

For the filling

½ cup + 2 tablespoons (5 oz) unsalted butter

⅔ cup (5 oz) soft light brown sugar

14 oz can condensed milk

For the topping

1 cup (5½ oz) bittersweet chocolate (see box, page 19)

¼ cup (1 oz) chopped pecans or brazil nuts

⅓ cup (2 oz) white chocolate (see box, page 19), chopped

2 tablespoons dried cranberries

2 tablespoons mini marshmallows (see box, page 19)

Preheat the oven to 375°F (190°C). Lightly oil an 8-inch (20 cm) square baking pan and line the base and sides with parchment paper.

Put the flours and sugars for the base into a food processor, and blend together. Add the butter, and pulse until the mixture starts to clump together. Tip the crumb mixture into the base of the prepared pan, and press very lightly to make an even layer. Bake the base in the oven for about 15 minutes, or until pale golden brown.

To make the filling, place the butter and sugar in a large nonstick pan over low heat, stirring until the butter melts and the sugar dissolves. Add the condensed milk, and bring gently to a boil, stirring continuously. Bubble gently for just 2 minutes, then remove from the heat. Spoon the caramel over the baked base, spreading it to the edges, and leave to cool for 30 minutes.

For the topping, melt the chocolate in a heatproof bowl set over a pan of just simmering water—don't let the bowl touch the water. Alternatively, you could use a microwave to gently melt the chocolate. Mix the remaining topping ingredients into the melted chocolate, and stir well. Spoon the mixture evenly over the caramel base. Leave to set in the fridge, and then cut it into squares to serve.

☐ **TO STORE:** The shortbread base will keep for 1 week stored in an airtight container.

✳ **TO FREEZE:** Wrap well, and freeze in an airtight container.

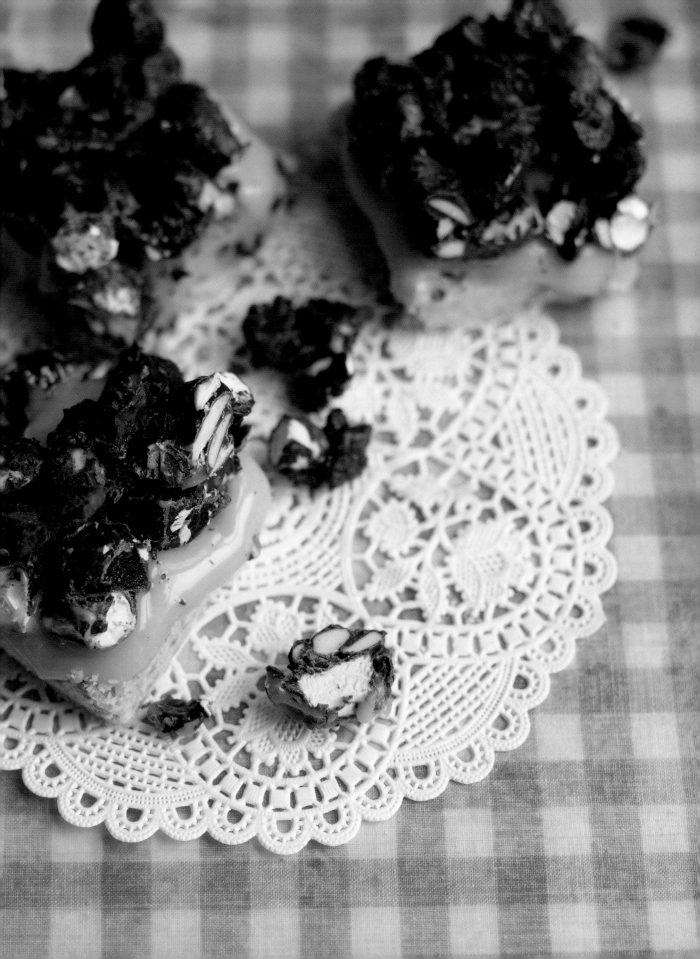

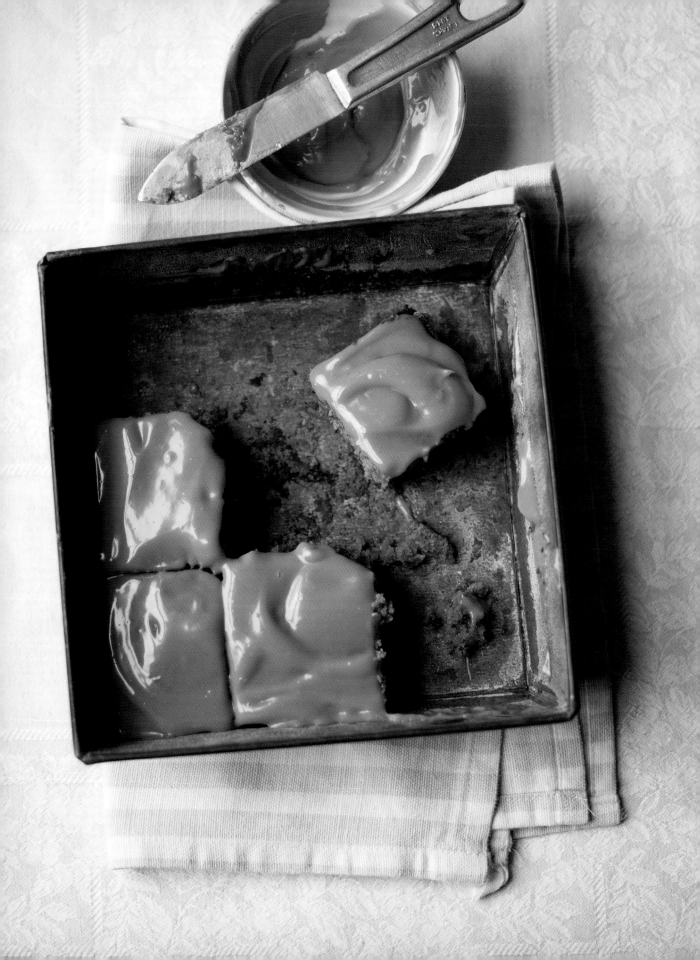

STICKY DATE, RUM & CARAMEL CAKE

A nice gooey caramel cake based on the British sticky toffee pudding recipe. I serve mine with ice cream or thick heavy cream. Medjool dates are best for this recipe, as they have a wonderful, melting, gooey texture.

MAKES: 6–8 SQUARES
PREPARATION: 10 MINUTES
BAKING: 20 MINUTES

---

vegetable oil, for oiling

1⅛ cups (6¼ oz) soft dates, pitted and roughly chopped

1 teaspoon baking soda

5 tablespoons dark rum or brandy

scant ½ cup (3½ fl oz) boiling water

1½ cups (6¼ oz) Gluten-Free Flour Mix B (see page 22)

1 teaspoon xanthan gum

1 teaspoon baking powder (see box, page 19)

6 tablespoons (3 oz) unsalted butter, softened

⅔ cup (5½ oz) dark brown sugar

2 large eggs, beaten, at room temperature

For the caramel sauce

14 oz dulce de leche, from a jar or can

Preheat the oven to 350°F (180°C). Oil a 7-inch (18 cm) square baking pan, and line base with parchment paper.

Put the dates, baking soda, rum, and boiling water into a small, heatproof bowl. Microwave on full power for 1 minute, and set aside to cool.

Sift the flour, xanthan gum, and baking powder together. Using a hand-held electric mixer, cream the butter with the sugar until it is light and fluffy, then gradually beat in the eggs. Fold in tablespoonfuls of the flour mixture, with alternate spoonfuls of the soaked dates and liquid, until the batter is evenly combined.

Pour the mixture into the prepared pan, and level the surface. Bake in the center of the oven for about 20 minutes, until firm and springy and a toothpick inserted into the center comes out clean.

To serve, spread the warm sponge cake with a layer of dulce de leche and cut into squares.

☐ **TO STORE:** The sponge cake will keep for 1 week (without the topping) stored in an airtight container. Top with the dulce de leche when you are ready to serve.

✱ **TO FREEZE:** Wrap well, and freeze in an airtight container. Defrost, warm for 10–15 seconds in the microwave, and spread with the dulce de leche when you are ready to serve.

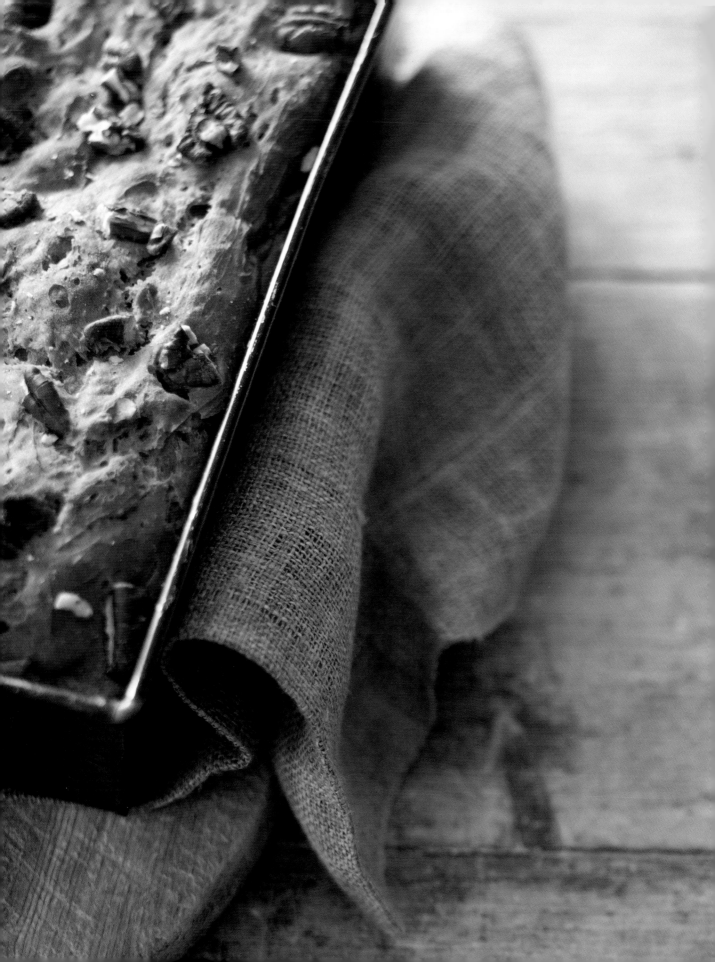

BREAD

CRISPY TORTILLA CHIPS

I love these! They are better than any you can buy, completely gluten-free, and really easy to make. It is best to cook them in small batches.

MAKES: ABOUT 20 CHIPS
PREPARATION: 10 MINUTES
COOKING: 10 MINUTES

¾ cup (3½ oz) Gluten-Free Flour Mix A (see page 22)

6 tablespoons fine cornmeal (see box, page 19)

¾ teaspoon xanthan gum

½ teaspoon baking powder (see box, page 19)

2 pinches of salt

about ½ cup (4 fl oz) warm water

cornstarch, for dusting

vegetable oil, for deep frying

salt and chili powder, for dusting

Place the flour, cornmeal, xanthan gum, baking powder, and salt in a bowl. Add enough warm water to form a soft dough.

Remove from the bowl, and knead well for 2–3 minutes, using a little dusting of cornstarch to prevent the dough from sticking to the work surface.

Divide the dough into 6–8 pieces—the smaller the pieces of dough, the easier it is to roll them out.

Dust a rolling pin well with cornstarch, and roll out a piece of dough as thinly as possible. Cut into small triangles.

Heat the vegetable oil to about 350°F (180°C) (check the temperature using a thermometer, or drop in a piece of bread—when it turns golden brown in 30 seconds the oil is ready), and deep-fry the tortillas in small batches until crisp on both sides.

Drain well on paper towels, and dust with salt and chili powder to serve.

☐ **TO STORE:** The chips will keep for up to 2 days stored in an airtight container.

✱ **TO FREEZE:** Not suitable.

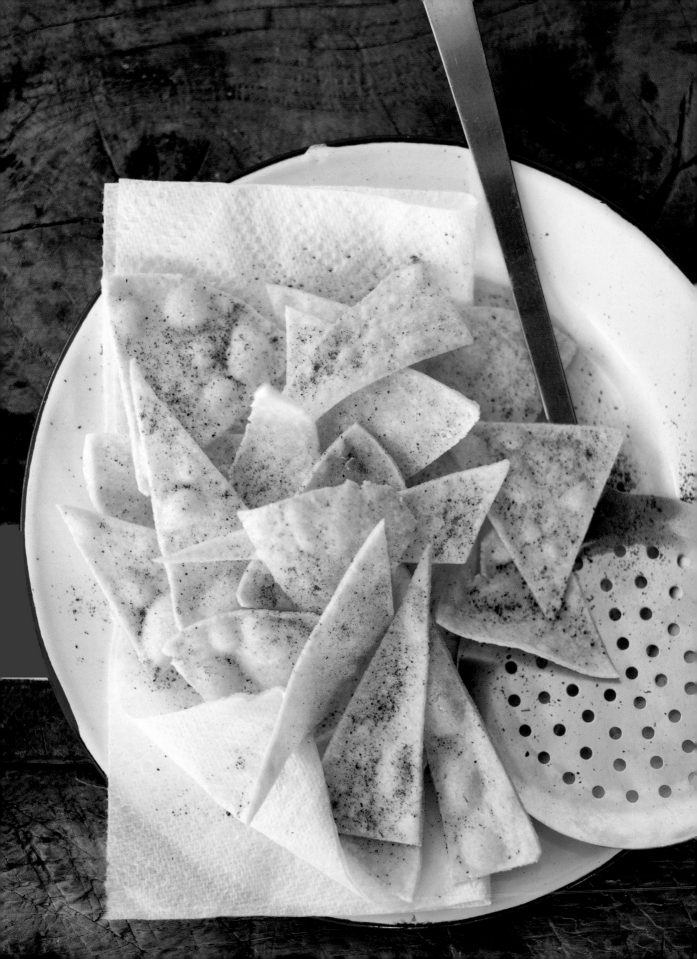

INDIAN-STYLE FLATBREADS

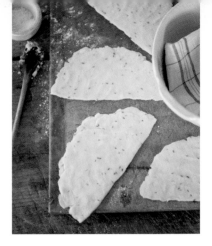

Here is a twist on the basic flatbread principle, delicious with all sorts of food, and great for dipping. I find it's best to leave them to cool completely to crisp up, then reheat them on a hot griddle or in a nonstick skillet for 30 seconds before eating.

MAKES: 6 BREADS
PREPARATION: 10 MINUTES
COOKING: 3–4 MINUTES FOR
   EACH BREAD

1⅛ cups (5½ oz) Gluten-Free
   Flour Mix A (see page 22)

½ teaspoon xanthan gum

3–4 pinches of salt (optional)

½ teaspoon whole cumin seeds

¼ teaspoon freshly ground
   black pepper

½ teaspoon baking powder
   (see box, page 19)

4 tablespoons olive oil

about ½ cup (4 fl oz) warm
   water

cornstarch, for dusting

olive oil, for brushing

Place the flour, xanthan gum, salt, cumin seeds, pepper, and baking powder in a bowl, and mix well. Add the oil and three-quarters of the warm water, and mix to form a wet dough. You may need to add a little more water to achieve this—aim for a slightly loose mix. Knead well on a board, using a little cornstarch to prevent the dough from sticking.

Cut the dough into 6 equal pieces. Roll out each piece into a circle, approximately 6 inches (15 cm) in diameter, as thin as you can—the thinner the better. Brush half of each circle with olive oil, then carefully fold in half, and press together to form a semicircle.

Heat a griddle pan or a 9-inch (23 cm) nonstick skillet over medium-high heat, then place the first bread in the pan with no oil. Cook for 2–3 minutes on each side, until the bread is slightly scorched on both sides. Remove from the pan, place on a wire rack, and brush lightly with olive oil. Repeat the process until all the breads are cooked, and serve immediately.

☐ **TO STORE:** These are best served immediately and I don't recommend storing them.

✱ **TO FREEZE:** Not suitable.

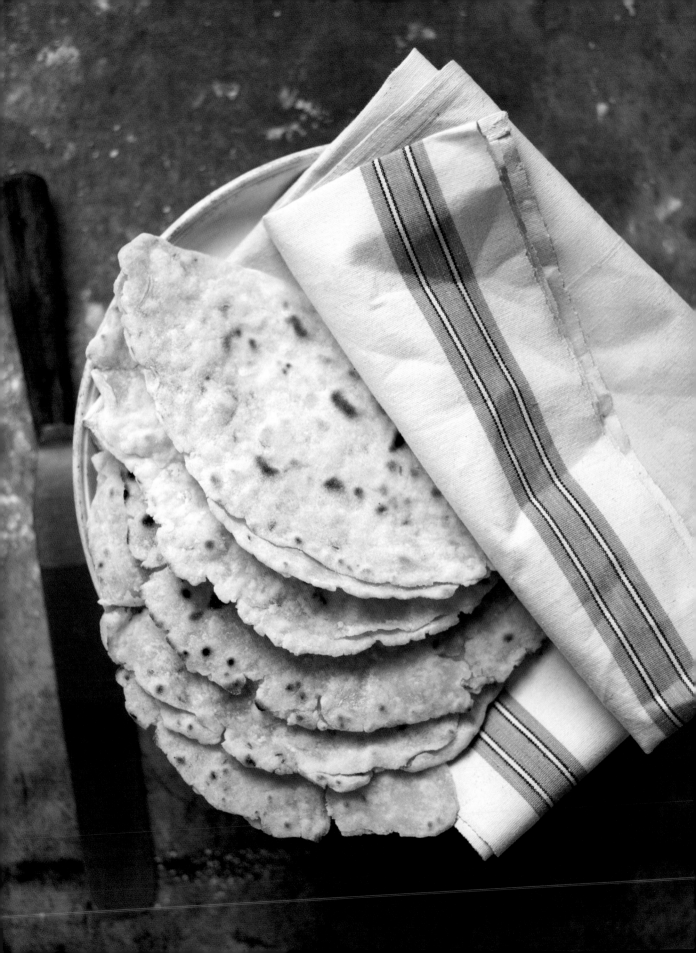

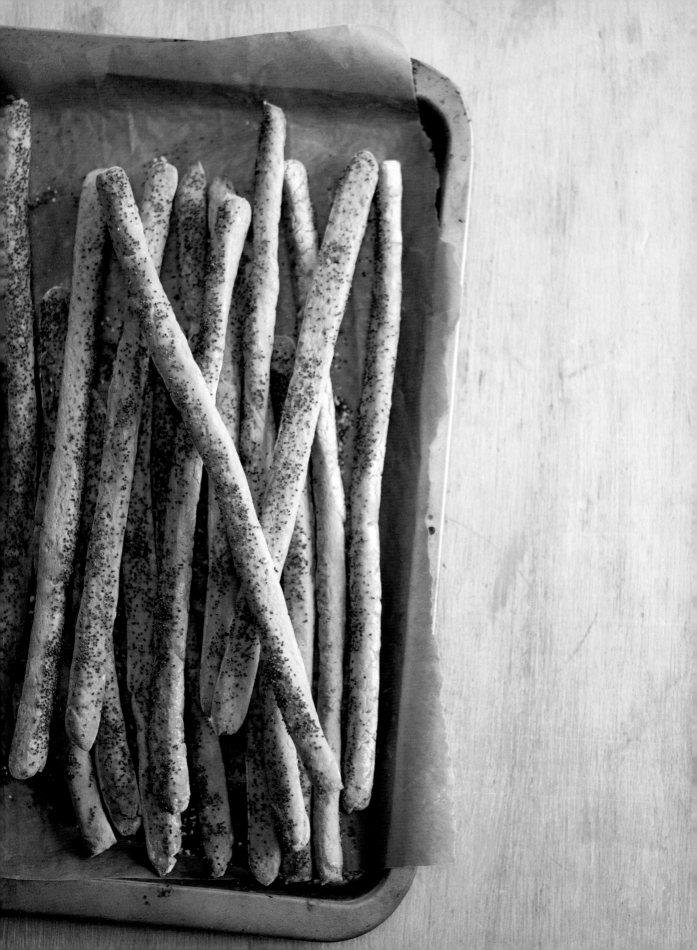

POPPY SEED BREADSTICKS

Easy to make and surprisingly addictive—good with dips and soups. Sesame, caraway, and fennel seeds also work well. You can make these by hand or in a breadmaker.

MAKES: 20 BREADSTICKS
PREPARATION: 30 MINUTES,
RISING TIME: 1 HOUR
BAKING: 10–15 MINUTES

3⅓ cups (11½ oz) Gluten-Free Bread Mix (see page 22)

2 teaspoons xanthan gum

1 teaspoon salt

2 teaspoons superfine sugar

¼-oz package active dry yeast

1 medium egg, at room temperature

scant cup (7½ fl oz) warm water

2 tablespoons olive oil

cornstarch, for dusting

vegetable oil, for oiling

1 egg, beaten, for brushing

1 tablespoon poppy seeds

If you are making the dough by hand, put the flour, xanthan gum, salt, sugar, and yeast into a large bowl, mix thoroughly, and make a well in the center. Stir the egg, water, and oil together in a bowl, and pour into the flour. Mix with a wooden spoon, and when the mixture tightens to form a dough, turn it out onto a board dusted with cornstarch. Flour your hands with cornstarch, and knead the dough for 5–10 minutes, until smooth.

Place the dough in a clean bowl, cover with oiled plastic wrap, and set it aside in a warm place to rise for about an hour, until doubled and puffy.

If you have a breadmaker, it's easier to control the variables and achieve a more consistent result. Simply pour the water, egg, and oil mixture into the pan first; add the flour mixture next, and sprinkle the yeast on top. Set the machine to "dough" and leave it to do the kneading and rising.

Preheat the oven to 425°F (220°C). Oil two baking sheets. Prepare your work surface with a large sheet of parchment paper dusted with cornstarch.

Turn out the dough and pat it into a rough rectangle about 10 × 6 × ½-inch thick (25 × 15 × 1cm thick). Cut it in half crosswise, and then into equal strips, like fingers. Handle the dough gently, and roll each strip with the palm of your hand into a long stick. (The thinner the sticks, the drier the texture.)

Transfer the breadsticks to a plate, brush with the beaten egg, and sprinkle with poppy seeds. Repeat for all the breadsticks, carefully lifting them onto the oiled baking sheet. Cover the line of breadsticks with oiled plastic wrap as you do this, and they will rise slightly at room temperature.

Bake the breadsticks for 10–15 minutes, until crisp and puffy. Allow to cool on the baking sheets.

These are best eaten fresh-baked, but you can refresh them in the microwave for a few seconds before serving.

☐ **TO STORE:** The breadsticks, if dried out well, will keep for up to 1 week in an airtight container.

✱ **TO FREEZE:** Freeze when cool, well wrapped and stored in an airtight container.

PARMESAN, SAGE, & ROAST GARLIC BISCUITS

I like savory biscuits, especially when spread with cold salted butter. I like them topped with guacamole, tahini, or even crab or shrimp cocktail.

MAKES: 10–12 BISCUITS
PREPARATION: 10 MINUTES
BAKING: 30–35 MINUTES

---

vegetable oil, for oiling

6 cloves garlic, unpeeled

2 cups (10¾ oz) Gluten-Free
   Flour Mix A (see page 22)

6 tablespoons (3 oz) margarine

pinch of salt

2 teaspoons xanthan gum

1 tablespoon baking powder
   (see box, page 19)

2 large eggs, beaten,
   at room temperature

2 teaspoons dried sage

½ cup (2 oz) Parmesan cheese,
   finely grated

½ cup (4 fl oz) 2% milk, warmed

cornstarch, for dusting

2% milk, for brushing

Preheat the oven to 400°F (200°C).

First, roast the garlic: wrap it in foil, and bake for 20 minutes. Remove the skins, and crush the creamy garlic.

Reduce the oven temperature to 350°F (180°C). Oil two baking sheets.

Place the flour, margarine, salt, and xanthan gum in a bowl, and rub together until you have the consistency of fine bread crumbs. Add the baking powder, eggs, sage, cheese, milk, and roasted garlic paste, and mix together to form a dough.

Dust a work surface with cornstarch and gently roll the dough out to about ½-inch (1 cm) thick. Using a 2-inch (5 cm) plain cookie cutter, stamp out 10–12 biscuits. Place on the baking sheets, brush with milk, and bake for 10–15 minutes.

Once baked, remove from the oven, and cool on a wire rack. Cut in half, and spread with salted butter to serve.

☐ **TO STORE:** The biscuits will keep for 2–3 days stored in an airtight container. They will dry out slightly after storing, so sprinkle with a little water, and then warm them through in a preheated oven at 400°F (200°C) for 5 minutes before serving.

✳ **TO FREEZE:** Wrap well, and freeze in an airtight container. The biscuits will dry out slightly after freezing, so once defrosted, sprinkle with a little water, and then warm them through in a preheated oven at 400°F (200°C) for 5 minutes before serving.

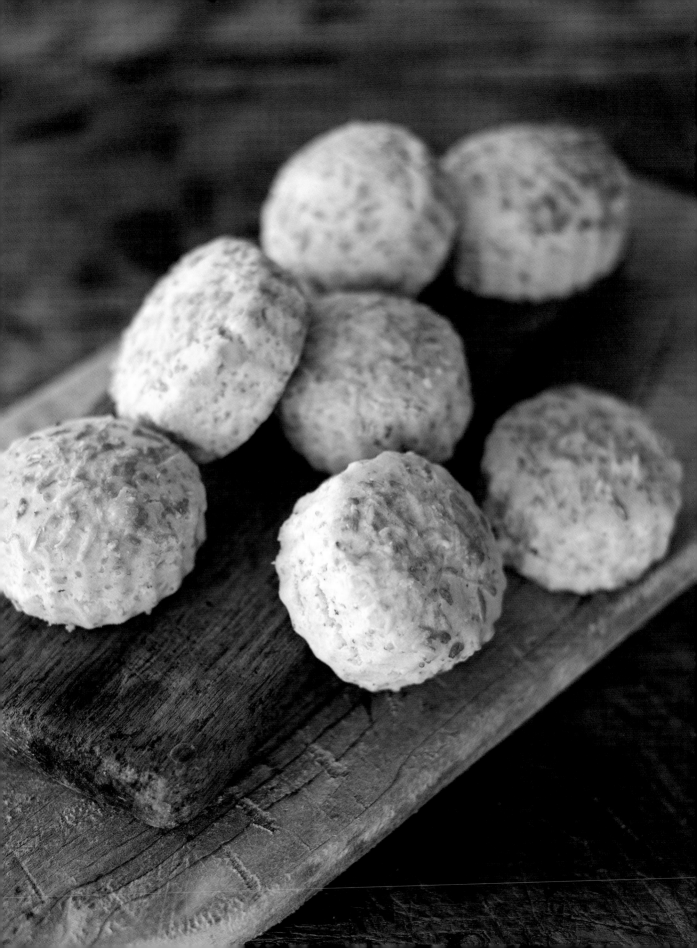

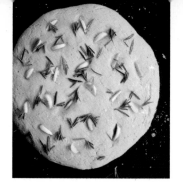

FOCACCIA

This recipe took seven attempts to get right—I wanted to achieve a light and spongy texture, and good flavor. As you will see, there is no salt in the mix. I find this tends to weaken the protein structure, giving you a less risen bread. I tend to stick to adding granular rock or sea salt to the top of the bread, along with olive oil, rosemary, and garlic cloves. I like to include vitamin C powder in this recipe, as I've found it really helps improve the structure of the bread. It is widely available from health food stores.

MAKES: ONE 12-INCH (30 CM) BREAD
PREPARATION: 20 MINUTES
BAKING: 15–20 MINUTES

---

vegetable oil, for greasing

2 × ¼-oz packages active dry yeast

generous 2 cups (17 fl oz) warm water

2 teaspoons superfine sugar

5¼ cups (18 oz) Gluten-Free Bread Mix (see page 22)

1 teaspoon xanthan gum

2 teaspoons baking powder (see box, page 19)

1 teaspoon vitamin C powder

2 egg whites

10 garlic cloves, halved

¼ cup olive oil

1 tablespoon sea salt

4–6 sprigs fresh rosemary

Oil a 12-inch (30 cm) nonstick pizza pan.

Whisk the yeast, water, and sugar together well, then cover and leave in a warm place for 15 minutes to activate.

Meanwhile, place the flour, xanthan gum, baking powder, and vitamin C powder into a bowl, and mix well.

When the yeast is frothy, whisk the egg whites until foamy. Pour the yeast mixture over the flour, add the whisked egg white, and bring together. Mix well, but do not overmix.

Spoon into the oiled pizza pan, cover lightly with plastic wrap, and press down lightly with your hands. Remove the plastic wrap.

Press the halved garlic cloves into the dough, and cover with a fresh piece of plastic wrap. Leave to rise in a warm place for 15–20 minutes, or until just doubled in height.

Meanwhile, preheat the oven to 425°F (220°C).

Once the dough has risen, carefully remove the plastic wrap, spoon on the oil, and sprinkle with the salt and rosemary. Bake for 15 minutes, or until well browned.

Remove from the oven, and cool on a wire rack. Slice into wedges to serve.

☐ **TO STORE:** The bread will keep for 1 day in an airtight container.

✱ **TO FREEZE:** Once cooled, wrap the bread well and freeze.

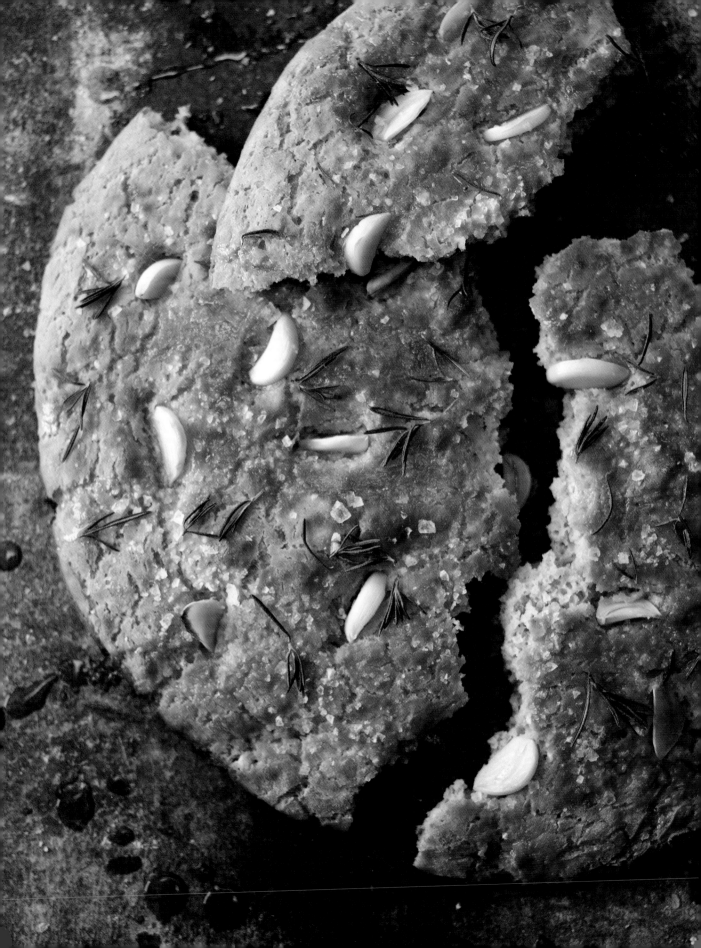

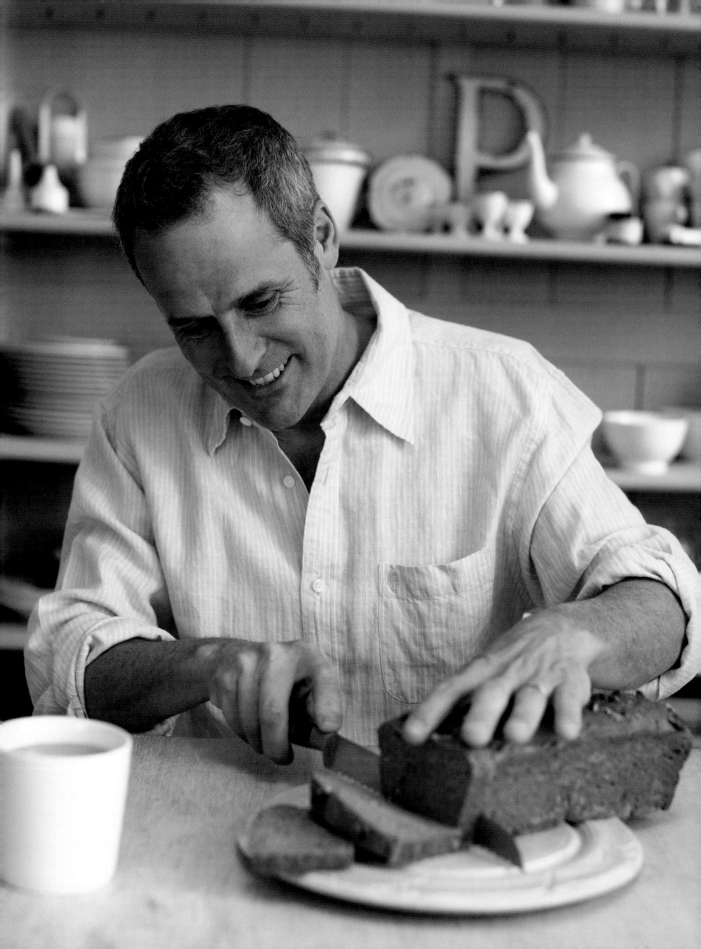

PECAN & MOLASSES BREAD

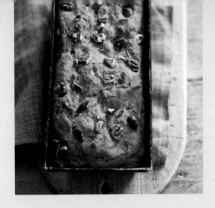

In *Seriously Good! Gluten-Free Cooking* I included only one recipe for bread, which contained chestnut flour. The people whose e-mails and letters I received loved it, but many of them had real trouble getting hold of chestnut flour. Not many stores stocked it, online stores had sporadic supplies, and it was quite expensive.

So here is another bread recipe; the texture is fairly light and airy, with a malt loaf background flavor, which comes from the molasses. It makes great toast.

MAKES: ONE 9 × 5-INCH
    (23 × 12 CM, 2 LB) LOAF
PREPARATION: 20 MINUTES
BAKING: 20–25 MINUTES

---

vegetable oil, for oiling

2 × ¼-oz packages active dry yeast

about 2 cups (16 fl oz) warm water

2 teaspoons superfine sugar

4¼ cups (14 oz) Gluten-Free Bread Mix (see page 22)

1 teaspoon salt

½ cup (2 oz) pecans, roughly chopped

2 teaspoons baking powder (see box, page 19)

2 teaspoons xanthan gum

1 tablespoon molasses

¼ cup (2 oz) margarine

1 large egg, beaten

Oil a 9 × 5-inch (23 × 12 cm, 2 lb) loaf pan.

Whisk the yeast, water, and sugar together well, then cover and leave in a warm place for 15 minutes to activate.

Meanwhile, place the flour, salt, nuts, baking powder, and xanthan gum together in a large bowl, and mix well. Place the molasses and margarine in a small nonstick pan, and warm through gently until the margarine has melted. Remove from the heat, and stir in the egg.

When the yeast mixture is ready, pour it over the flour mixture, and add the molasses mixture. Mix well with a wooden spoon, but do not go mad, or the mixture will tighten considerably.

Spoon the mixture into the oiled loaf pan, cover with plastic wrap, and press the mixture into the pan, then lift off the plastic wrap. Cover lightly with a clean piece of plastic wrap, and leave to rise in a warm place for 20 minutes.

Meanwhile, preheat the oven to 425°F (220°C).

Once the dough has risen, bake the loaf for 20 minutes, until well risen and nicely colored. Remove from the pan and cool on a wire rack.

☐ **TO STORE:** Once cooled, wrap well in plastic wrap, or store in an airtight container for up to 3 days.

✻ **TO FREEZE:** Wrap well, and freeze in an airtight container. Defrost to room temperature before eating.

RUM-SOAKED BABAS WITH APRICOT GLAZE

Babas are yeasty fruit buns soaked in rum syrup, which used to be all the rage at dinner parties. Serve with vanilla ice cream, or for a real treat, my favorite—clotted cream (which is available at specialty stores and online).

MAKES: 12 BABAS
PREPARATION: 30 MINUTES
RISING TIME: 45 MINUTES
BAKING: 15–20 MINUTES

For the babas

vegetable oil, for oiling

⅔ cup (5 fl oz) warm water

2 × ¼-oz packages active dry yeast

6 tablespoons (3 oz) superfine sugar

1¾ cups (7 oz) Gluten-Free Flour Mix B (see page 22)

1 teaspoon xanthan gum

2 teaspoons baking powder (see box, page 19)

½ cup (3½ oz) golden raisins

¼ cup (2 oz) currants

¼ cup (2 oz) margarine

1 teaspoon glycerin

2 teaspoons vanilla extract

3 large egg whites, at room temperature

cornstarch, for dusting

For the syrup

1 cup (8 oz) superfine sugar

4–6 tablespoons rum

6 tablespoons apricot jelly

Generously oil a 12-cup nonstick muffin pan.

Mix the warm water, yeast, and 2 teaspoons of the sugar. Whisk well, cover with plastic wrap, and set aside.

In a separate bowl, place the flour, xanthan gum, baking powder, remaining sugar and fruit, and mix really well.

Melt the margarine in a small nonstick pan and add the glycerin and vanilla to the pan.

Whisk the egg whites until soft peaks form.

Pour the yeast mixture over the flour and fruit, then add the melted margarine mixture, and finally the egg whites. Fold together well, but do not go mad.

Spoon the mixture into the prepared muffin pans, press down lightly with fingers dusted with cornstarch, and cover with plastic wrap. Leave in a warm place to rise to the top of the pans (about 45 minutes in a warm place).

When risen, preheat the oven to 400°F (200°C). Bake the babas for 10–15 minutes, until well-risen and lightly colored. Remove from the oven, and cool in the pans for 5–10 minutes.

Make the syrup by placing the sugar, rum, and 1 scant cup (7½ fl oz) cold water in a small pan and simmer until the sugar has dissolved. Once dissolved, dip the babas in, one by one, and turn over several times so they soak up the hot syrup. Once well soaked, carefully lift out with a slotted spoon, and place on a wire rack to drain well and cool.

Heat the apricot jelly and 1 tablespoon water until well mixed, and, using a pastry brush, coat the babas thoroughly with the glaze, and allow to cool again.

☐ **TO STORE:** The babas will keep for up to 2 days, before soaking and glazing, stored in an airtight container. Soak and glaze as above before serving.

✱ **TO FREEZE:** Wrap well when cool, and freeze, before soaking and glazing. Defrost for 1 hour, then soak and glaze.

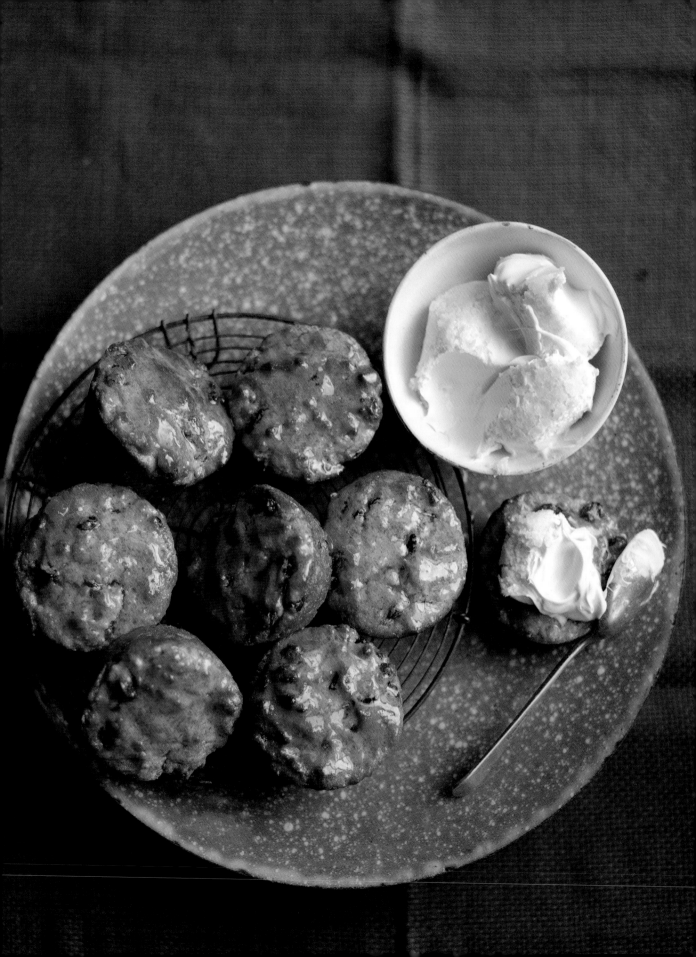

GOLDEN RAISIN BRIOCHE LOAF

One of the nicest breads to eat, especially for breakfast. This recipe comes very close to the real thing, with a lovely flavor and texture.

MAKES: ONE 9 × 5-INCH
    (23 × 12 CM, 2 LB) LOAF
PREPARATION: 15 MINUTES
RISING TIME: 1 HOUR OR SO
BAKING: 25–30 MINUTES

---

vegetable oil, for oiling

½ cup (4 fl oz) 2% milk

1 extra large egg, at room
    temperature

2½ cups (11½ oz) Gluten-Free
    Flour Mix A (see page 22)

1 teaspoon xanthan gum

1 teaspoon salt

2 tablespoons superfine sugar

¼-oz package active dry yeast

⅞ cup (7 oz) unsalted butter,
    chilled and cubed

½ cup (3 oz) golden raisins

Lightly oil a 9 × 5-inch (23 × 12 cm, 2 lb) loaf pan.

In a small pan, warm the milk with ⅓ cup (2½ fl oz) water, add the egg and beat lightly.

Put the flour, xanthan gum, salt, sugar, and yeast in a food processor, and pulse to mix. Add the butter, and process briefly to cut the butter into the mixture. Leave the butter in very small pieces; you don't want it to go to bread crumbs.

Empty the contents of the food processor into a large bowl. Make a well in the center, and add the golden raisins and milk and egg mixture. Fold the ingredients together briefly; it will still be a bit lumpy.

Spoon the mixture into the prepared pan. Cover with plastic wrap, and pat down to flatten nicely, then lift off the plastic wrap, and cover with a clean piece of plastic wrap.

Leave to rise in a warm place for 1 hour.

When risen, preheat the oven to 400°F (200°C). Bake for 25–30 minutes, or until well risen and dark golden. Remove from the oven and eat while warm and fresh.

☐ **TO STORE:** The brioche will keep for up to 2 days, stored in an airtight container.

✲ **TO FREEZE:** Slice when cold, double wrap in plastic wrap, and freeze in an airtight container. Remove individual slices of the bread, and toast from frozen as required.

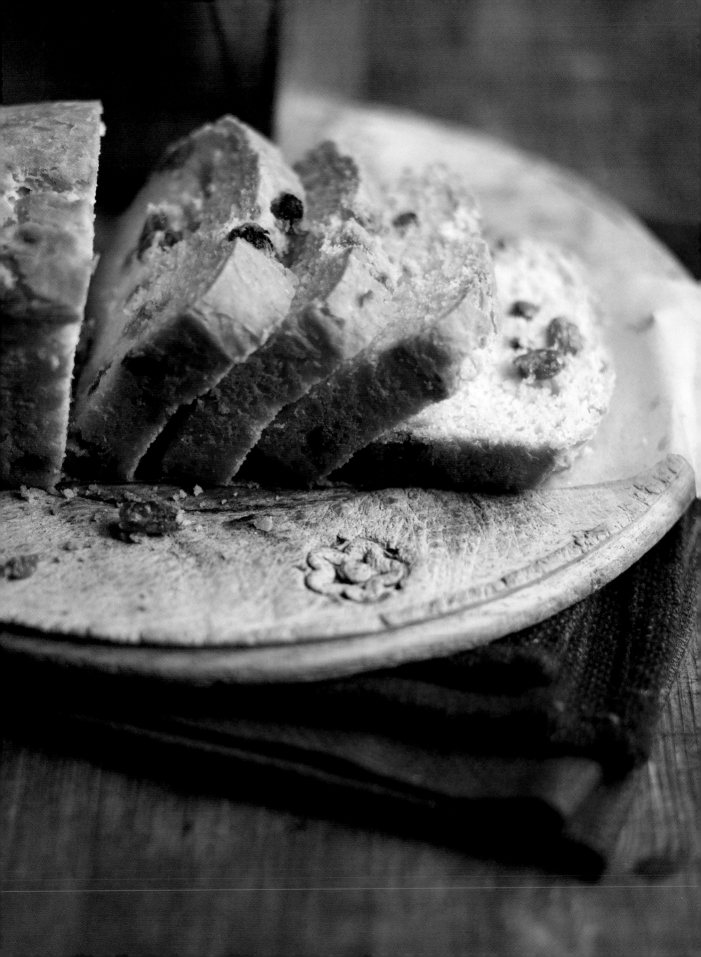

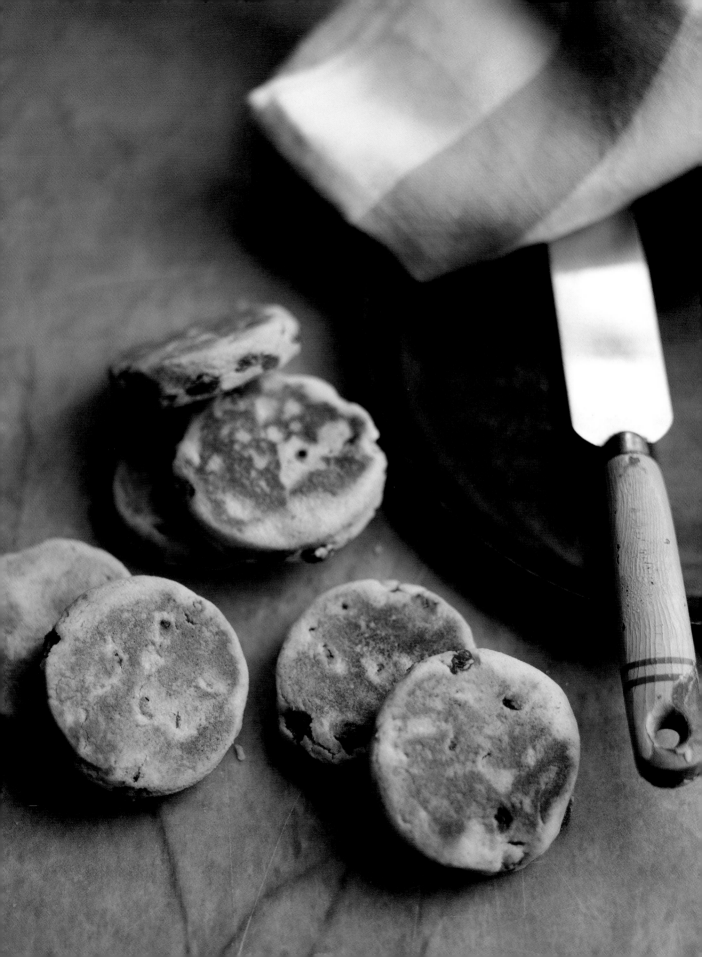

WELSH CAKES

The original basic recipe for these cakes came from my stepchildren's grandmother, Joan. The cakes are so good, and really simple to make; in fact I still have the original recipe she gave me about 10 years ago.

The gluten-free version has a slightly more crumbly texture than usual, but I think it works fine this way. If you like, replace half the margarine with lard—this adds a deeper flavor and also makes a shorter texture.

MAKES: ABOUT 10–12 CAKES
PREPARATION: 10 MINUTES
COOKING: 15–20 MINUTES

1¾ cups (8 oz) Gluten-Free Flour Mix A (see page 22)

1 teaspoon pumpkin pie spice

7 tablespoons (3½ oz) margarine

½ teaspoon xanthan gum

½ teaspoon baking soda

1 teaspoon glycerin

6 tablespoons superfine sugar

½ cup (3 oz) golden raisins

1 large egg, beaten

cornstarch, for dusting

superfine sugar, for sprinkling

Place the flour, spice, margarine, xanthan gum, and baking soda in a bowl, and rub through gently with your fingers until you have the texture of fine bread crumbs. Next add the glycerin, sugar, golden raisins, and egg, and mix together lightly until a soft dough is formed.

Roll the dough out on a work surface dusted with cornstarch to a thickness of ¼-inch (5 mm). Using a 3-inch (8 cm) plain cookie cutter, stamp out 10–12 little cakes.

Heat a griddle pan or 9-inch (23 cm) nonstick skillet over medium heat. Add 4 cakes to the pan, and cook for 2–3 minutes on each side, until lightly colored and puffy.

Once cooked, remove from the pan, and sprinkle with superfine sugar. Serve warm, spread with butter.

☐ **TO STORE:** The cakes will keep for 2 days stored in an airtight container. Warm through for 10 seconds in the microwave before serving.

✱ **TO FREEZE:** Once cooked, freeze in an airtight container. Defrost for 1 hour, and warm through for 10 seconds in the microwave before serving.

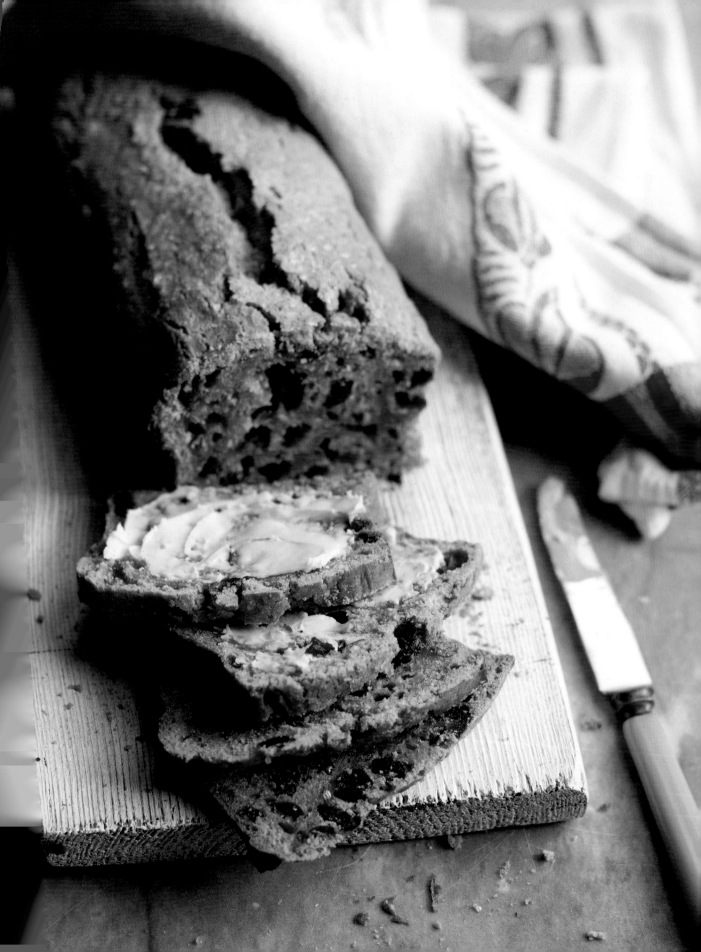

CHRISTMAS CHESTNUT & CRANBERRY BREAD

This makes a great alternative if you are not too keen on Christmas cake. Chestnut purée really helps the texture of the end result here. And you can bake it in advance, as it freezes really well.

Serve it spread generously with butter—brandy butter is especially appropriate at Christmas!

MAKES: ONE 9 × 5-INCH (23 × 12 CM, 2 LB) LOAF
PREPARATION: 15 MINUTES
BAKING: 50–60 MINUTES

---

vegetable oil, for oiling

⅔ cup (4½ oz) potato flour

1 cup (3½ oz) tapioca flour

½ teaspoon ground nutmeg

½ teaspoon ground cinnamon

2 teaspoons baking powder (see box, page 19)

1 teaspoon xanthan gum

1 cup (8 oz) unsweetened chestnut purée

3 large eggs, at room temperature

7 tablespoons (3½ oz) margarine

⅔ cup (5½ oz) superfine sugar

⅔ cup (3½ oz) dried cranberries

1 tablespoon light brown sugar

Preheat the oven to 325°F (160°). Oil and line the base of a 9 × 5-inch (23 × 12 cm, 2 lb) loaf pan.

Sift the flours together into a medium bowl with the spices, baking powder, and xanthan gum.

In a food processor, process the chestnut purée, then add the eggs one at a time, and process until smooth.

Cream the margarine and sugar together in a large bowl, using a hand-held electric mixer, then add the chestnut mixture; don't worry if it curdles. Next fold in the flour mixture with a large metal spoon, and finally, stir in the cranberries.

Spoon the mixture into the prepared pan, and sprinkle with the light brown sugar. Bake in the center of the oven for about 50 minutes, or until the top is golden brown and a toothpick inserted into the center comes out clean. Leave to cool in the pan for 10 minutes, then turn out onto a wire rack.

Serve fresh, sliced and buttered.

☐ **TO STORE:** The bread will keep for up to 2 days stored in an airtight container.

✳ **TO FREEZE:** Cool and slice, then wrap well in plastic wrap, and freeze. Remove slices of the bread as required, defrost for 1 hour, and serve with butter.

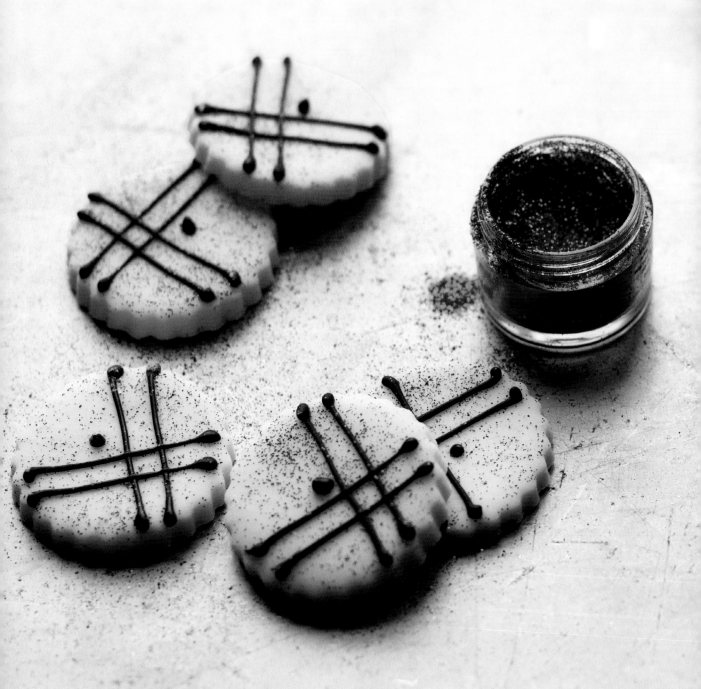

DESSERTS & SWEET TREATS

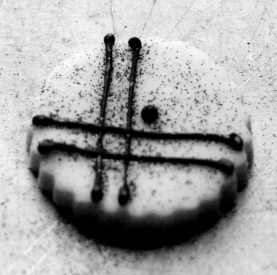

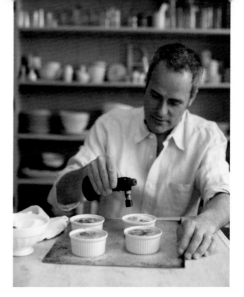

CHEAT'S RASPBERRY CRÈME BRÛLÉE

This is a recipe from a friend of mine, Paul. He serves it in his pub, and it always goes down incredibly well! It is really easy and takes out all the hassle involved in the traditional method. Use clear ramekins if possible so you can see the raspberries inside.

SERVES: 6
PREPARATION: 15 MINUTES

scant cup (7 oz) ready-made custard (see box, page 19)

½ cup (4 oz) mascarpone cheese

½ cup (4 oz) crème fraîche

2 tablespoons (1 oz) superfine sugar

2½ cups (10 oz) fresh or frozen raspberries

3 tablespoons superfine sugar, for glazing

Put the custard, mascarpone cheese, crème fraîche, and 2 tablespoons superfine sugar into a large bowl, and gently whisk together until the mixture thickens. Divide the raspberries equally between 6 small ramekins (approximately ½ cup, [4 oz]) and then carefully spoon the creamy mixture over the fruit. Tap the dishes on the worktop so the creamy mixture covers the raspberries, and chill well in the fridge for about 2 hours.

When you are ready to serve, unless you have a cooks' blowtorch, preheat the broiler to high. To finish, carefully sprinkle ½ tablespoon superfine sugar over each one, and place briefly under the hot broiler to caramelize, or glaze the tops with the blowtorch. Serve immediately.

☐ **TO STORE:** Store in the fridge for 2–3 hours, if needed, before glazing the tops.

✳ **TO FREEZE:** Not suitable.

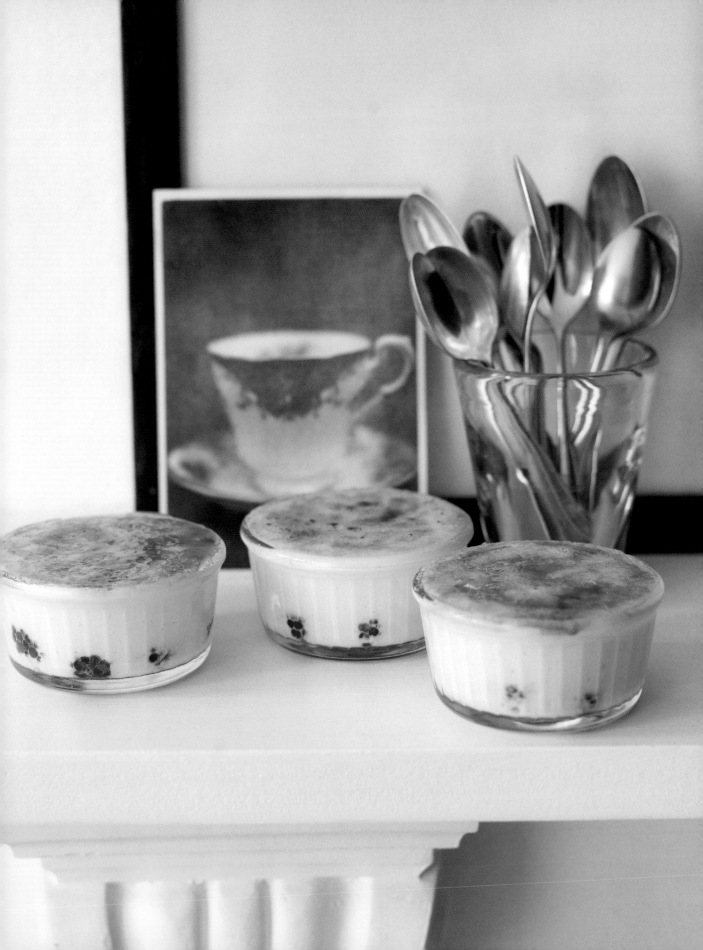

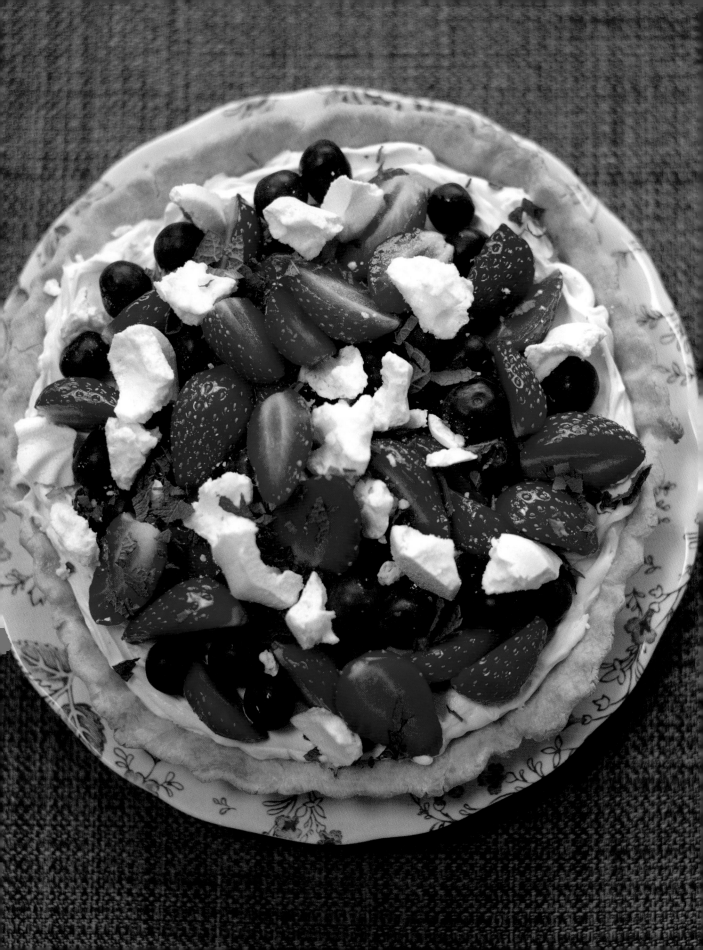

STRAWBERRY TART WITH CRUSHED MERINGUE & MINT

This is a great summer treat, and any combination of fresh seasonal fruit will work well. Just pile high, top with crushed meringue, and drizzle with the yogurt sauce. For best results, remove from the fridge 30 minutes before eating, so the fruit is not too cold.

MAKES: ONE 8-INCH
   (20 CM) TART
PREPARATION: 10 MINUTES,
   PLUS CHILLING
BAKING: 25 MINUTES FOR
   THE TART CRUST

For the tart crust

vegetable oil, for oiling

1¾ cups (8 oz) Gluten-Free Flour
   Mix A (see page 22)

1 teaspoon xanthan gum

1 tablespoon superfine sugar

½ cup (4 oz) cooking margarine

1 large egg, at room temperature

cornstarch, for dusting

For the filling

1¼ cups (9 oz) ready-made
   custard (see box, page 19)

1 cup (8 oz) mascarpone cheese

1 cup (5 oz) strawberries, halved

¾ cup (3½ oz) blueberries

1 tablespoon chopped fresh mint

½ cup (2 oz) meringue cookies
   (see box, page 19), crumbled

For the yogurt sauce

scant cup (7 oz) plain yogurt

4 tablespoons maple syrup

2 tablespoons chopped mint

Preheat the oven to 350°F (180°C). Oil an 8-inch (20 cm) fluted tart pan with removable bottom, and line base with parchment paper.

Mix the flour with the xanthan gum and sugar, then add the margarine, rubbing in with your fingers until the mixture looks like fine bread crumbs. Beat the egg, reserve a little to brush the crust with during baking, then add the rest of it to the mixture, along with 1 tablespoon water, and mix well to make a dough. Keep an eye on the texture; you may need to add another tablespoon water so it's nice and soft.

Roll out the pastry on a work surface dusted with cornstarch, to a 9-inch (23 cm) circle. Lift the pastry carefully into the pan, and press it into the base and up the sides. Shape the pastry into the sides with your thumbs, but don't make it too thin. Line with a layer of parchment paper and dried beans, then bake blind for 15 minutes. Carefully lift out the parchment paper with the beans, brush the base and sides of the pastry with the remaining beaten egg, and return it to the oven for another 10 minutes. Remove, and set aside to cool.

Make the filling: beat the custard and mascarpone together in a medium bowl, using a hand-held electric mixer. Spread this mixture into the baked and cooled crust. Top with the strawberries and blueberries. Mix the mint into the crumbled meringues, and pile on top. Chill the tart for 30 minutes.

Combine all the sauce ingredients in a small pitcher, and chill. Serve the tart no longer than 2 hours after filling it, or it will go soggy. Serve chilled wedges of the tart with the sauce.

☐ **TO STORE:** The unfilled tart crust can be stored for up to 24 hours in an airtight container.

✳ **TO FREEZE:** Not suitable.

MY MOM'S ORANGE GELATIN, PEACH & WHITE CHOCOLATE CHEESECAKE

I have to hold my hand up here; yes, this is my mom's recipe—she has been making it for years. It's so simple, and the end result is very good indeed, so I just had to steal the recipe!

MAKES: ONE 7-INCH (18 CM) ROUND CHEESECAKE
PREPARATION: 20 MINUTES, PLUS CHILLING

For the cheesecake

vegetable oil, for oiling

about 8 (8 oz) gluten-free cookies or shortbread (try the recipe on page 23)

⅓ cup (2 oz) white chocolate (see box, page 19)

For the filling

½ package (1½ oz) orange gelatin dessert

1 15-oz can peaches, drained

1 cup (8 oz) cottage cheese

1¼ cups (10 fl oz) heavy whipping cream

For the topping

2 fresh peaches, sliced

½ cup (2 oz) white chocolate (see box, page 19), grated

Oil a 2½-inch (6 cm) deep, 7-inch (18 cm) round, nonstick cake pan with a removable bottom, and line base with parchment paper.

Place the shortbread in a food processor, and process to crumbs. Melt the chocolate in a heatproof bowl in the microwave, or over a pan of simmering water—don't let the bowl touch the water. Add the melted chocolate to the crumbs, and blitz again until the mixture starts to clump together. Press the crumb mixture into the cake pan, without packing it down too much, and then chill really well.

Next, make up ½ package (45g, 1½ oz) orange gelatin dessert. Set aside to cool.

In a blender or food processor, blend the drained peaches until you have a thick purée, then add the cottage cheese, heavy cream, and cooled gelatin dessert. Blend until smooth—probably 15 seconds at the most.

Pour the filling over the base, and return to the fridge for at least 1 hour to set.

When set, remove from the fridge, and top with the fresh, sliced peaches. Sprinkle with the grated white chocolate. The cheesecake should be served within 2–3 hours of adding the topping.

☐ **TO STORE:** The cheesecake base can be stored for up to 24 hours in an airtight container in the fridge.

✳ **TO FREEZE:** Not suitable.

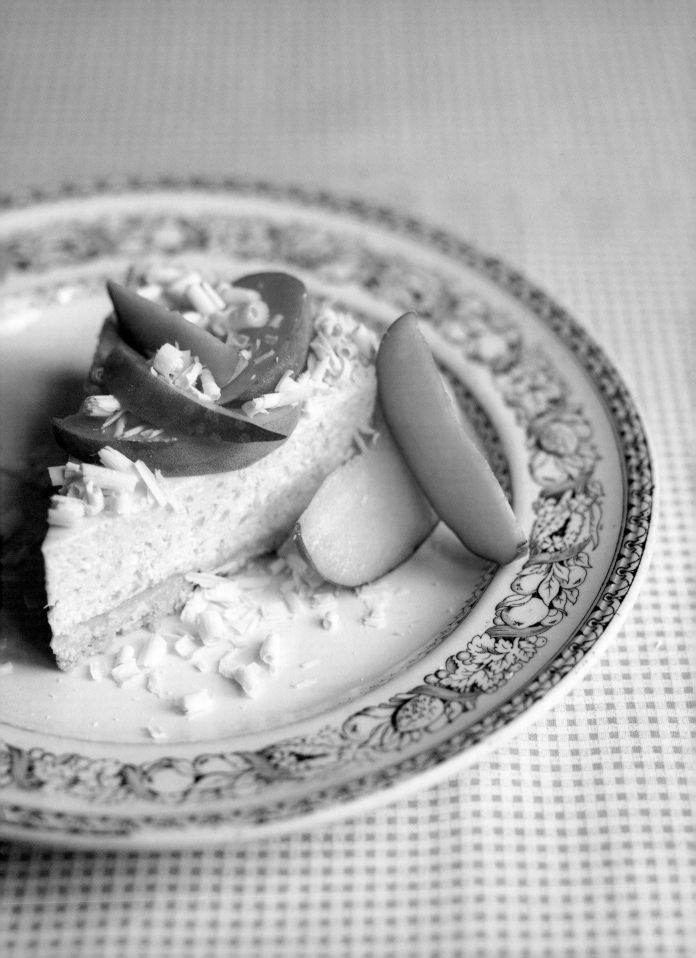

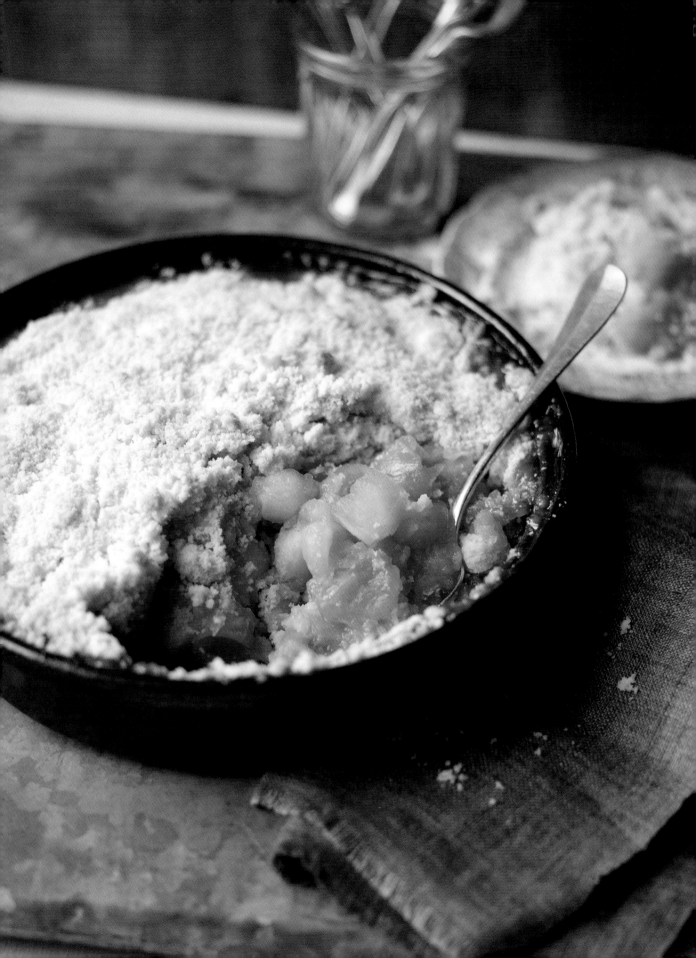

CARAMEL APPLE CRUMBLE

I love caramel apples, and this is a great way to include their delicious flavor in a dessert! You can use either McIntosh, Granny Smith, or Jonathan varieties. Their tart flavor, coupled with caramel, makes a great combination. I like to serve this with ice cream or custard.

SERVES: 4–6
PREPARATION: 15 MINUTES
BAKING: 25–30 MINUTES

¾ cup (6 oz) soft light brown sugar

zest and juice of 2 large lemons

3 tart apples, peeled, cored and roughly chopped

For the topping

2¼ cups (10¾ oz) Gluten-Free Flour Mix A (see page 22)

½ cup + 2 tablespoons (5 oz) unsalted butter, chilled

6 tablespoons superfine sugar

Preheat the oven to 400°F (200°C).

Place the sugar in a large saucepan over high heat, and bring to a boil. The sugar will melt to form a clear liquid. Boil until it turns a pale amber color. This will take about 10 minutes.

Add the lemon zest and juice and the apples to the pan, and cook for 5–6 minutes. Place in a 9½-inch (24 cm) baking dish.

For the topping, place the flour and butter in a food processor, and blitz until smooth. Just pulse in the sugar; do not overwork. Carefully spoon the topping over the cooked apples.

Bake for 25–30 minutes, or until well browned and cooked. Serve warm.

☐ **TO STORE:** Not suitable.

✳ **TO FREEZE:** Not suitable.

CHOCOLATE CHEESECAKE

No baking book would be complete without a baked cheesecake—it is just the thing to satisfy a sweet tooth. Just remember not to overbake it—keep it nice and wobbly to ensure a soft, melting center.

MAKES: ONE 7-INCH (18 CM)
ROUND CHEESECAKE
PREPARATION: 15 MINUTES,
PLUS OVERNIGHT CHILLING
BAKING: 20 MINUTES,
PLUS 1 HOUR SETTING

___

For the base

vegetable oil, for oiling

scant cup (4½ oz) rice flour

2 tablespoons superfine sugar

2 tablespoons soft brown sugar

6 tablespoons (3 oz) unsalted
butter, cubed

For the filling

¾ cup (3½ oz) bittersweet
chocolate (see box, page 19)

1¾ cups (14 oz) light or
medium-fat cream cheese

scant ½ cup (3½ oz) superfine
sugar

1 teaspoon vanilla extract

scant cup (7 oz) Greek yogurt

2 large eggs, at room
temperature

For the topping

½ cup (4 oz) frozen forest berry
mix, defrosted and drained

2 tablespoons cherry jelly

Preheat the oven to 350°F (180°C), and set a shelf just below the center. Lightly oil a 2½-inch (6 cm) deep, 7-inch (18 cm) cake pan with a removable bottom, and line base with parchment paper.

Put the flour and sugars for the base into a food processor, and blend together. Add the butter, and process until the mixture forms fine crumbs, and then starts to clump together. Tip the crumb mixture into the base of the prepared pan, and press lightly to make an even layer. Put the base into the oven for about 15 minutes, or until baked and pale golden brown. Remove the pan and stand it in a roasting pan.

To make the filling, melt the chocolate in a heatproof bowl, in the microwave or over a pan of simmering water, and set aside. In a large bowl, beat the cream cheese, sugar, and vanilla with a hand-held electric mixer, then add the yogurt and the eggs, one at a time. Mix until well blended, then add the melted chocolate to the bowl, and mix until smooth. Pour the filling over the base in the cake pan, and shake gently to level.

Bake for 20 minutes: it will have just set around the edges but still be wobbly in the middle. Turn the oven off, and leave the cheesecake inside to cool slowly for 1 hour; it will continue to cook—and this helps to avoid the top cracking—so don't open the oven door.

Refrigerate until ready to serve, preferably overnight.

To serve, loosen the edges of the cheesecake with a spatula, and unmold onto a plate. Crush the fruits lightly, combine with the jelly, and spoon on top.

☐ **TO STORE:** The cheesecake will keep for up to 2 days in an airtight container in the fridge.

✱ **TO FREEZE:** Freeze, uncovered, without the fruit topping. Once frozen, wrap well in plastic wrap and foil, and return to the freezer. Top with the fruit once defrosted.

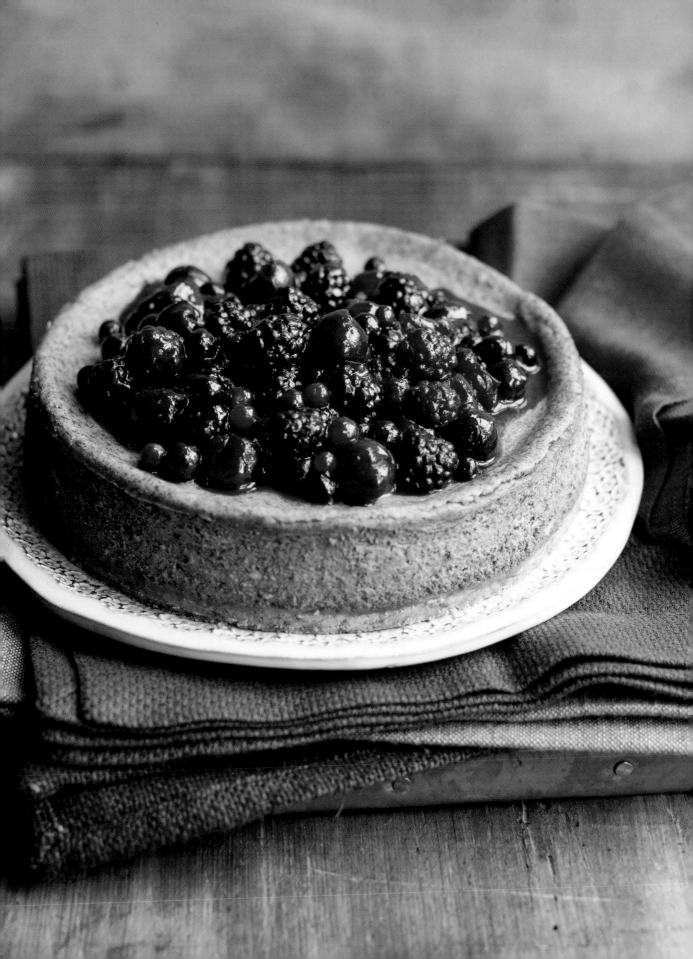

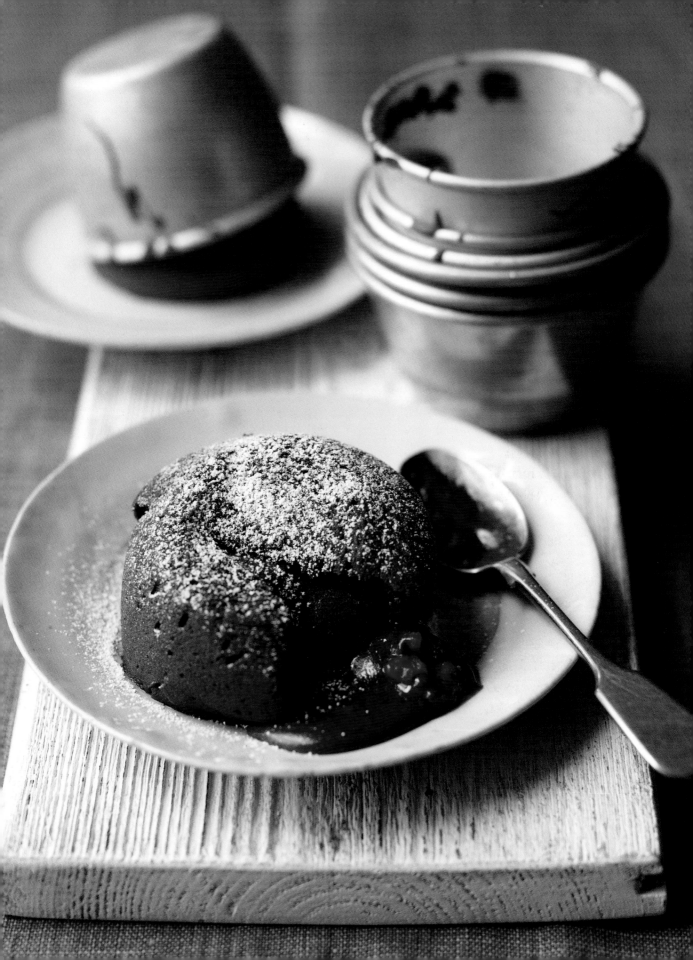

HOT CHOCOLATE FONDANT PUDDINGS WITH RASPBERRIES

This is a classic, simple dessert that never fails to impress. The individual puddings can be made up to 24 hours in advance, stored in the fridge, and then baked when you are ready. Remember, don't overbake them, and serve with cream or ice cream.

   I like to use semi-thawed frozen raspberries for these puddings, as they produce more delicious juice than fresh berries.

SERVES: 6
PREPARATION: 20 MINUTES
BAKING: 12–15 MINUTES

vegetable oil, for oiling

2 cups (12½ oz) bittersweet chocolate (see box, page 19)

¼ cup (2 oz) unsalted butter, softened

6 tablespoons superfine sugar

generous ½ cup (6 oz) condensed milk

4 extra large eggs, beaten, at room temperature

1 teaspoon vanilla extract

generous ⅔ cup (3 oz) Gluten-Free Flour Mix A (see page 22)

½ cup (4 oz) frozen raspberries, semi-thawed

sifted confectioners' sugar, to serve

Place a large baking sheet in the oven and preheat it to 400°F (200°C). Oil 6 individual ramekins (approximately 5 fl oz), and cut circles of parchment paper to line the bases.

   Melt the chocolate in a heatproof bowl in the microwave, or over a pan of simmering water—don't let the bowl touch the water—and set aside. Cream the butter and the sugar together in a large bowl, using a hand-held electric mixer, until light and fluffy. Slowly whisk in the condensed milk. Gradually beat in the eggs and the vanilla.

   Stir in the melted chocolate, and finally, add the flour, mixing until smooth.

   Divide half the chocolate mixture evenly between the ramekins. Layer the raspberries equally over the chocolate. Finally, spoon the remaining chocolate mixture evenly over the raspberries.

   Place the ramekins on the hot baking sheet in the oven, and bake for 12–15 minutes, until puffed and risen. Remove from the oven, and run a knife around the edge of the puddings to unmold onto a serving plate. Dust with confectioners' sugar, and serve immediately.

☐ **TO STORE:** Not suitable.

✳ **TO FREEZE:** Not suitable.

STEAMED GOLDEN SYRUP SPONGE PUDDING WITH CUSTARD

A classic childhood pudding, just right for a cold winter's day—soft and crumbly, with lots of syrup. It will also reheat perfectly, gently heated after being left to cool for a couple of hours.

SERVES: 4–6
PREPARATION: 15 MINUTES
COOKING: 50–55 MINUTES

For the pudding

melted butter, for greasing

3 large eggs, at room temperature

finely grated zest of 1 lemon

½ cup (4 oz) superfine sugar

4 tablespoons golden syrup

scant cup (4½ oz) Gluten-Free Flour Mix A (see page 22)

½ teaspoon baking powder (see box, page 19)

1 teaspoon xanthan gum

1 teaspoon glycerin

scant ½ cup (3½ fl oz) vegetable oil

For the custard

2½ cups (20 fl oz) 2% milk

scant ½ cup (2 oz) custard powder (see box, page 19)

superfine sugar or golden syrup, to taste

Grease a 1-quart heatproof glass bowl with the butter. Place a steamer pan on the stove, and half fill with water. Check that the bowl fits snugly inside the steamer with the lid on.

In a stand mixer on high speed, beat the eggs, lemon zest, and superfine sugar until very thick and mousse-like.

Using a spoon dipped in hot water, place the golden syrup in the greased bowl. Mix together the flour, baking powder, and xanthan gum really well in a separate bowl. Combine the glycerin and oil together in a cup. Remove the bowl from the mixer, and sprinkle in the flour mixture. Add the oil mixture, and gently whisk it all together.

Pour the mixture into the greased glass bowl; it will be over three-quarters full at this point. Cover tightly with buttered foil. Put it into the boiling steamer and place the lid on, then steam for 50–55 minutes. Keep an eye on the boiling water—you may need to top it up with water from the kettle.

Once cooked, the sponge will have risen to the top of the bowl. Carefully remove from the steamer, and leave for 5 minutes to set.

Meanwhile, make the custard by mixing a quarter of the milk with the custard powder in a bowl. Bring the rest of the milk to a boil in a small nonstick saucepan. Once boiling, carefully pour in the cold milk and custard powder mixture, while gently whisking continuously. The milk should thicken immediately, and just boil. Remove from the stove, and add the sugar or syrup to taste; bear in mind you will have plenty of sweetness from the pudding itself.

Remove the foil from the pudding, and turn out onto a large bowl or plate. Serve immediately with plenty of hot custard.

☐ **TO STORE:** Not suitable.

✳ **TO FREEZE:** Freeze the cooled pudding in the bowl, covered with foil. Defrost for 1–2 hours. To reheat, cover with plastic wrap, and cook in the microwave in 30-second bursts.

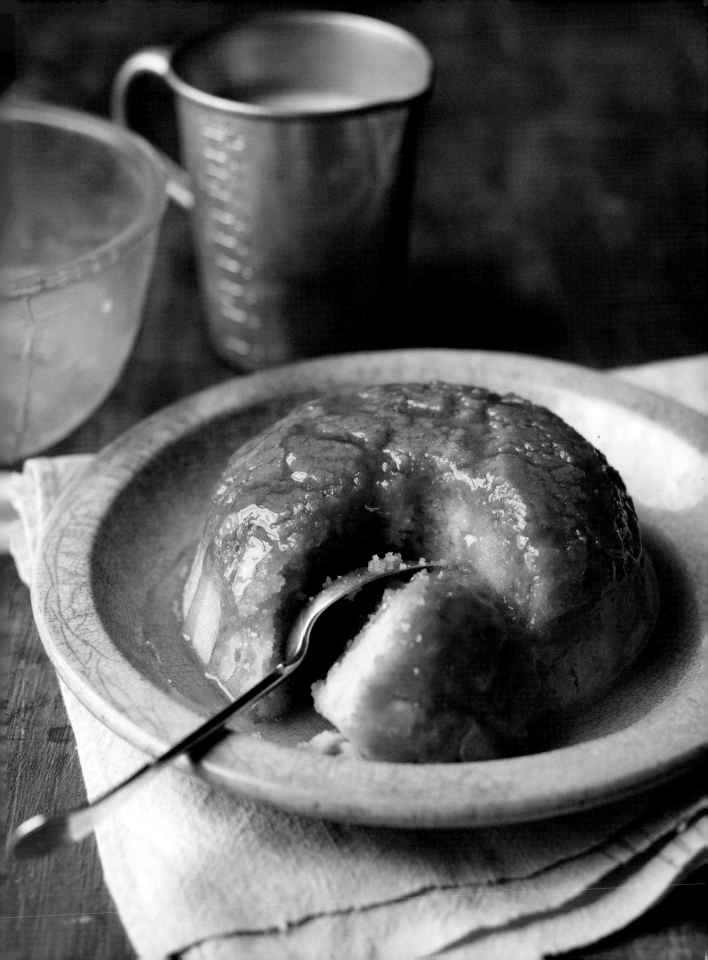

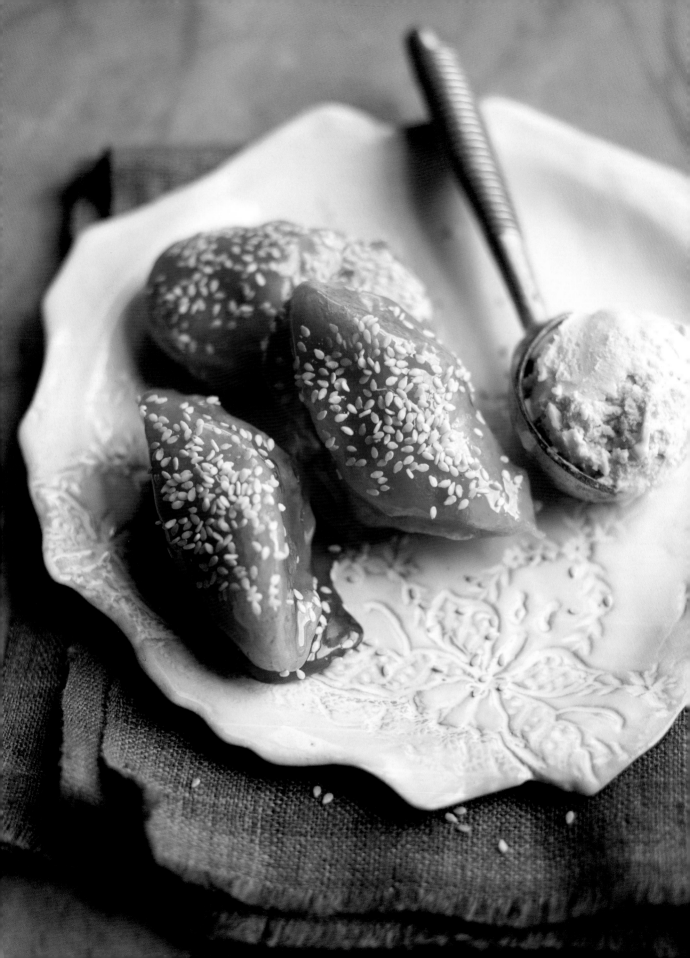

SESAME SEED BANANA FRITTERS

Bananas deep-fried in a light Chinese-style batter and dipped in crisp caramel—fab! I like to toss them in the traditional coating of sesame seeds, along with some crushed Brazil nuts.

SERVES: 4
PREPARATION: 20 MINUTES
COOKING: 30 MINUTES

¾ cup (3½ oz) Gluten-Free Flour Mix A (see page 22)

1½ teaspoons baking powder (see box, page 19)

1¼ cups (10 fl oz) vegetable oil, for frying

4 medium bananas

2 tablespoons sesame seeds

1 tablespoon crushed, toasted Brazil nuts (optional)

scant cup (7 oz) superfine sugar

Mix the flour with the baking powder. Gradually stir ⅔ cup (5 fl oz) cold water into the flour to make a thick, smooth paste; it should be a little thicker than heavy cream, and you may need to adjust the amount of water slightly to achieve a coating batter.

Organize yourself with a couple of metal slotted spoons, paper towels for draining, and the bowl of batter ready, so you can use it immediately.

Heat the oil in a medium, deep saucepan: it's hot enough when a cube of bread sizzles and turns golden in a few seconds.

Slice the bananas into quarters, and dip a few at a time into the batter. Use a slotted spoon to drain the excess batter off, and lift the pieces into the hot oil (a frying basket will make this easier). Deep-fry the bananas in batches, for about 1½ minutes each. With a clean slotted spoon, turn them in the oil until pale golden, and drain on paper towels. When you have cooked all the bananas, prepare the caramel.

Mix the sesame seeds with the Brazil nuts, if using, and set aside. Melt the sugar with 4 tablespoons cold water in a small, heavy-bottomed saucepan over low heat. Stir gently, and only when all the sugar crystals are dissolved, stop stirring and allow it to boil. Bubble until the mixture turns a dark golden caramel color—about 10 minutes. Remove from the heat.

Use two wooden skewers to pick up the banana pieces and dip them into the hot caramel sauce. Roll one side in the sesame seeds and transfer them to a sheet of parchment paper set over a wire rack. Leave the banana fritters briefly for the caramel to harden, then serve immediately.

A note of caution: Because of the high temperatures reached by the oil and the sugar, you will need to keep a careful watch during all the stages, and the pans should not be left unsupervised. I wouldn't recommend making this with children, but they will enjoy the end result!

☐ **TO STORE:** Not suitable.

✳ **TO FREEZE:** Not suitable.

CHOCOLATE PEPPERMINT FONDANT CREAMS

A favorite from childhood, which I've given a grown-up twist—simple, good fun, and tasty.

MAKES: APPROXIMATELY 18
PREPARATION: 15 MINUTES,
PLUS 1 HOUR SETTING TIME

---

6 tablespoons (4 oz) condensed milk

2 cups (8 oz) confectioners' sugar, sifted

3–4 drops natural peppermint extract

confectioners' sugar, for dusting

¼ cup (1 oz) bittersweet chocolate (see box, page 19)

edible glitter (see box, page 19)

Pour the condensed milk into a large bowl, and gradually mix in the confectioners' sugar to make a smooth paste. Next add the peppermint extract. Knead the paste until it is smooth and firm. The fondant should keep its shape; add a little more confectioners' sugar if it seems too soft or too sticky.

Roll the fondant out on a work surface dusted with confectioners' sugar to ¼-inch (5 mm) thickness, and then cut into rounds with a 1¼-inch (3 cm) cookie cutter. Place the creams on parchment paper and leave in a cool place to set—this will take about 1 hour.

Melt the chocolate in a heatproof bowl in the microwave or over a pan of simmering water, and set aside. Decorate the peppermint creams with the melted chocolate by drizzling it over in lines, or dip into the melted chocolate to coat one half.

Sprinkle a little edible glitter over to give them a professional finish.

☐ **TO STORE:** Allow the chocolate to set, and store in an airtight container for up to 1 month.

✱ **TO FREEZE:** Not suitable.

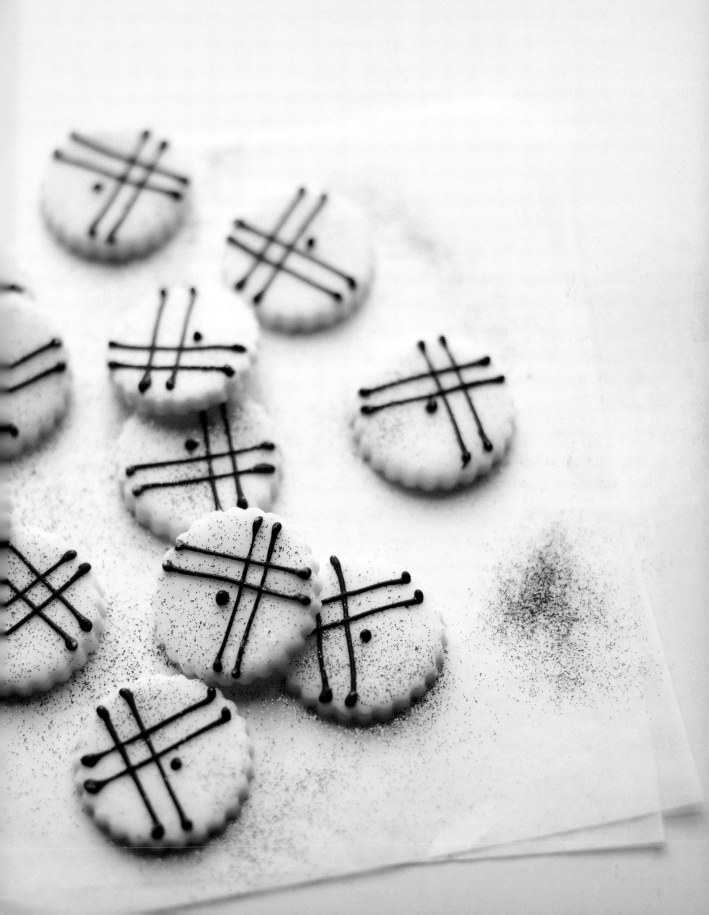

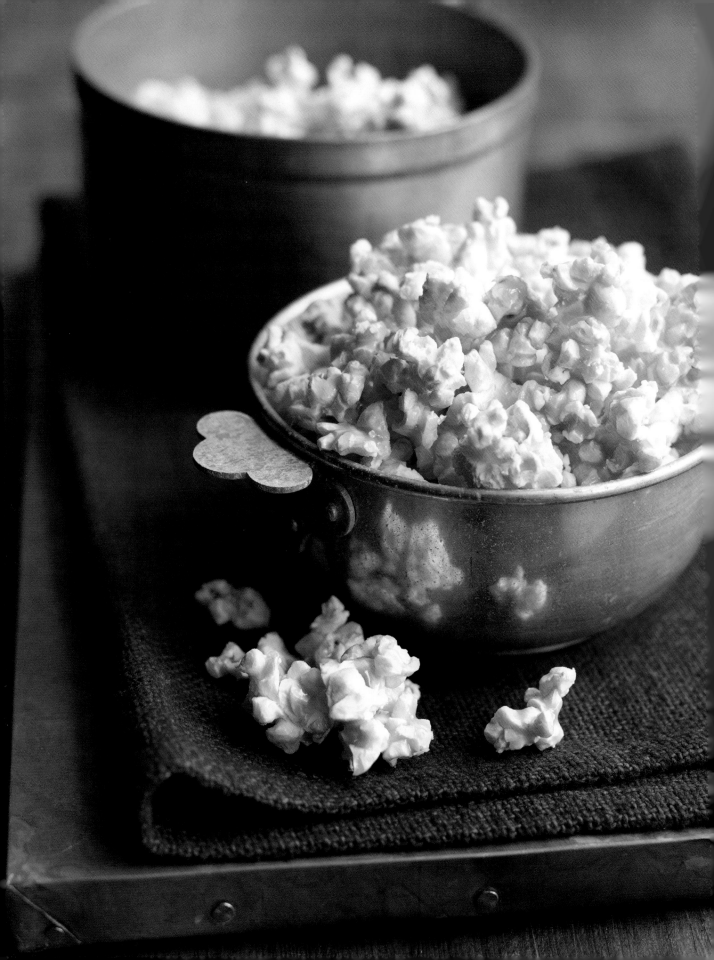

SALTED CARAMEL POPCORN

I love this! Salted caramel popcorn has become all the rage over the past year or two. I find that the microwave salted variety works the best—it's easy and foolproof. If you can't get hold of microwave popcorn, this also works with regular popcorn kernels.

SERVES: 2–3
PREPARATION: 5 MINUTES
COOKING: 5–15 MINUTES

3½ oz package salted microwave popcorn or ½ cup (3½ oz) popcorn kernels plus 1 tablespoon vegetable oil

scant ½ cup (3½ oz) superfine sugar

2 tablespoons (1 oz) unsalted butter

For microwave popcorn: Cook the popcorn according to the manufacturer's instructions, and tip into a large bowl. Reject any hard kernels.

For popcorn kernels: Heat the oil in a large pan, and add the popcorn kernels. Cover tightly with a lid, and heat gently, shaking the pan until all the corn is popped. The trick is to listen, and when the popping slows right down (after approximately 8–10 minutes), remove the pan from the heat, and tip the popcorn into a large bowl.

Spread the sugar over the base of a wide, heavy-bottomed pan, over medium heat, and keep an eye on it until it begins to melt and caramelize. Swirl the pan to make an even, dark golden liquid; watch carefully, and take it off the heat before it gets too dark, or it will taste bitter. Carefully whisk in 1 tablespoon water and the butter, and stir to a smooth, rich caramel.

Trickle the caramel onto the popcorn in the bowl, using two forks to pull the clumps apart, and coat the popcorn as it cools.

☐ **TO STORE:** The popcorn will keep well in an airtight container for a couple of days.

✳ **TO FREEZE:** Not suitable.

DIRECTORY

CELIAC SOCIETIES

Your national celiac society can provide more information about celiac disease, put you in touch with local groups and keep you informed about events relating to celiac disease.

CANADA

Canadian Society of Intestinal Research
855 West 12th Avenue
Vancouver, BC V5Z 1M9
Tel: 604 875 4875
www.badgut.com

Canadian Digestive Health Foundation
1500 Upper Middle Road, Unit 3
PO Box 76059
Oakville, ON L6M 3H5
Tel: 905 829 3949
www.cdhf.ca

Canadian Celiac Association
5170 Dixie Road, Suite 204
Mississauga, Ontario L4W 1E3
Tel: 905 507 6208
www.celiac.ca

Fondation Quebecoise de la Maladie Coeliaque
4837 rue Boyer, Bureau 230
Montreal, Quebec H2J 3E6
Tel: 514 529 8806
www.fqmc.org

UNITED STATES

Celiac Disease Foundation
13251 Ventura Blvd Ste 1
Studio City, CA 91604
Tel: 818 990 2354
www.celiac.org

Celiac Sprue Association
P.O. Box 31700
Omaha, NE 68131-0700
Tel: 402 558 0600
www.csaceliacs.org

Gluten Intolerance Group
31214 124th Ave SE
Auburn, WA 98092-3667
Tel: 253 833 6655
www.gluten.net

American Celiac Society Dietary Support Coalition
PO Box 23455
New Orleans, LA 70183-0455
Tel: 504 737 3293
www.americanceliacsociety.org

National Foundation for Celiac Awareness (NFCA)
224 South Maple Street
Ambler, PA 19002
Tel: 215 325 1306
www.celiaccentral.org

American Celiac Disease Alliance
2504 Duxbury Place
Alexandria, VA 22308
Tel: 703 622 3331
americanceliac.org

GLUTEN-FREE PRODUCTS

If you are unable to find gluten-free products at your local supermarket or health food store, try the following online suppliers.

CANADA

eatit.ca Canada's Online Organic Store
603 Wall Street
Winnipeg, MB R3G 2T5
Tel: 204 772 2136
www.eatit.ca

Cream Hill Estates
9633 rue Clément
LaSalle, QC H8R 4B4
Tel: 514 363 2066
www.creamhillestates.com

El Peto Products
www.elpeto.com

Duinkerken Foods
57 Watts Avenue
Charlottetown, PEI C1E 2B7
Tel: 902 569 3604
www.duinkerkenfoods.com

Go Bio Foods
RR 1
Acton, ON L7J 2L7
Tel: 519 853 2958
www.gobiofood.com

UNITED STATES

Ener-G Foods
5960 First Avenue South
PO Box 84487
Seattle, WA 98124-5787
Tel: 206 767 6660
www.ener-g.com

Gluten Free
www.glutenfree.com

Gluten Free Mall
www.glutenfreemall.com

Gluten Solutions
www.glutensolutions.com

Mixes from the Heartland
www.mixesfromtheheartland.com

Shop Organic
www.shoporganic.com

Aunt Gussie's
141 Lanza Avenue, Building 8
Garfield, NJ 07026
Tel: 973 340 4480
www.auntgussies.com

Schär
1050 Wall Street West, Suite 203
Lyndhurst, NJ 07071
www.schar.com/us/

Allergy Free Shop
8803 SW 132 Street
Miami, FL 33176
Tel: 305 254 2828
www.allergyfreeshop.com

Gluten-Free Trading Co.
3116 S Chase Avenue
Milwaukee, WI 53207
Tel: 414 747 8700
www.food4celiacs.com

INDEX

ACKNOWLEDGMENTS

There are so many people I would like to thank. This sort of book takes many people to help, check, recheck and publish.

Firstly, thank you to Kyle Cathie for being brave and re-signing me—hope you like it.

Thanks to Jenny Wheatley, for bringing it all together and making some sense of all the experiments; Jacqui Caulton, for the fab design; Annie Rigg and Rachel Wood, for making all the food look great; Wei Tang, spot-on as usual; Elanor Clarke and Gemma John, lovely job; and Jane Bamforth, for helping in all the areas I had forgotten about.

A big thank you to Tara Fisher for the simply wonderful photos, and for getting me to smile at the right time. Bea Harling, good friend and without whose help I don't know what I would have done when I was stuck!

Thanks to all the girls at Coeliac UK who checked and rechecked; Amy Peterson, Kathryn Miller and Jo Archer, whose help and advice has been invaluable.

To John Rush, my close friend and agent, and Luigi Bonomi—the best around by far.

Finally, Fernie—you make everything I do possible.

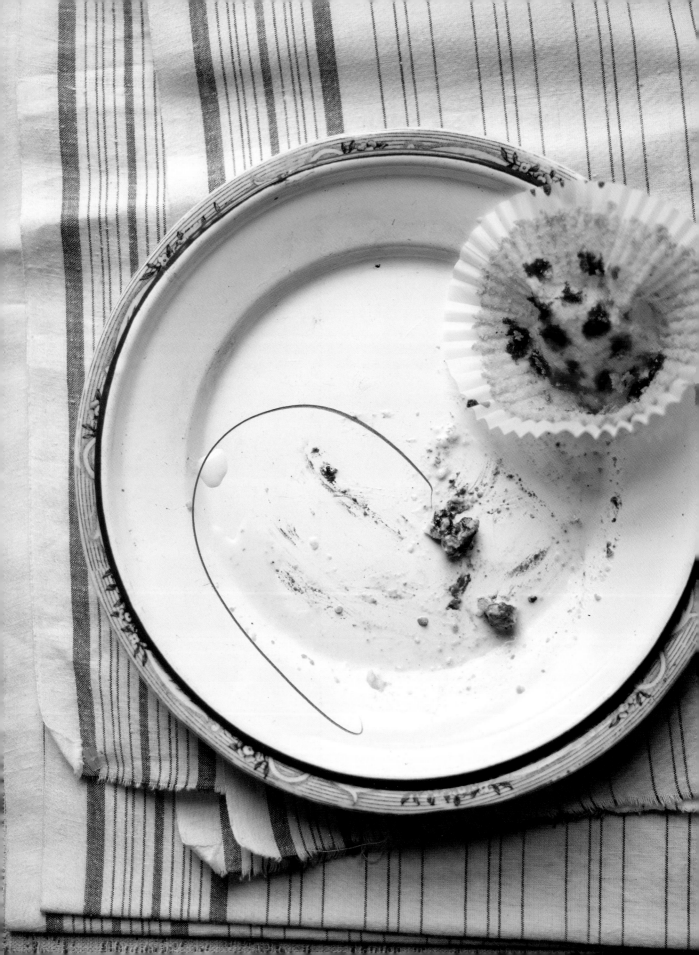